リハビリテーション英語の基本用語と表現

編著者
清水雅子，服部しのぶ

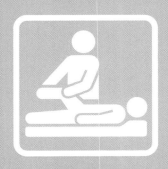
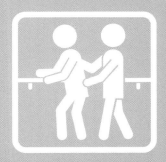

Essential Terms
And Expressions
For Rehabilitation

MEDICAL VIEW

Essential Terms and Expressions for Rehabilitation
(ISBN 978–4–7583–0441–2 C3047)

Editors: Masako Shimizu and Shinobu Hattori

2015. 2. 1　1st ed.

©MEDICAL VIEW, 2015
Printed and Bound in Japan

Medical View Co., Ltd.
2–30 Ichigaya–honmuracho, Shinjuku–ku, Tokyo 162–0845, Japan
E-mail　ed@medicalview.co.jp

刊行にあたって

　近年，リハビリテーションの専門領域は，身体的・精神的障害をもつ人々の社会復帰を目指して，他の医療分野・医学との連携を深めながら，著しい発展を遂げています。さらに，国際交流の機会も増え，日本はリハビリテーションの実践モデル国として期待され，海外から協力を要請される時代となってきました。

　このような状況に合わせて，リハビリテーションに関わる人々が，専門英語の運用能力を総合的に習得できるようにと考えて，この小辞典は編纂されました。そのために，専門領域の基本用語だけでなく，治療の場面で用いられる英語表現も併せてPart 1〜4で構成しました。

　Part 1はリハビリテーションの基本事項に関する用語，Part 2は症状と疾患・障害の名称，Part 3は人体の各部位の名称と機能の用語を掲載しています。それらは項目別に分類され，重要語は太字で，一般用語は青字で示されています。

　Part 4では患者を指導する英文例を，ADLおよび主要な疾患別に，実際のリハビリテーションの場面を想定して作成しました。英文を前後関係の中で理解し，覚えることが重要です。またコラムでは，語源や英語と日本語の違いなどを通して，専門英語の特徴を知り，関心を深めてほしい，と希望しています。本書を常時携帯し，反射的に英語が口をついて出てくるまで活用され，さらに，それぞれの専門領域の英語へと発展されることを願っております。

　なお，本書の出版にあたり，適切なご助言とご尽力をいただきましたメジカルビュー社編集部 江口潤司氏に心よりお礼申し上げます。

2015年1月

編著者

〈凡例〉

1. Part 1〜3は用語集です。左欄に英語，右欄に日本語が記載されています。

    表記上の指定は下記の通りです。

    ①各トピック毎に分類され，トピックの中ではアルファベット順に並んでいます。

    ②同義語は「; 」で併記されています。日本語訳が異なる場合は英語に対応して「；」で併記されています。

    　例：lateral position; side-lying position　　側臥位；横臥位

    ③日本語訳が複数ある場合は「, 」で併記されています。

    　例：depression　　引き下げ，下制，低下

    ④親子関係の語句は1字下げで表記されています。

    　例：position　　　　　　　　　　肢位, 体位
    　　　anatomical position　　解剖学的肢位

    ⑤〔　〕は省略可能を示します。

    　例：心電図検査〔法〕＝「心電図検査」または「心電図検査法」

    ⑥（　）は言い換えを示します。

    　例：ずり(肘)這い　＝「ずり這い」または「肘這い」

    ⑦《　》は注釈を示します。

    ⑧**太字**は重要語，青文字は一般英語での言い換え表現を示します。

2. Part 4は会話表現集です。英文が青文字で示され，その下に日本語訳が黒文字で示されます。

3. 索引は，日本語は五十音順，英語はアルファベット順で配列されています。訳語は併記していませんので，自己診断にご利用ください。

目次

Part 1 Rehabilitation Terms リハビリテーションの基本英単語 1

1. Positions, Ranges of Motion, Activities and Gaits 肢位・体位・姿勢・関節可動域・動作・歩行 ……… 2

- **1-1.** Positions and Postures　肢位・体位・姿勢 ……… 2
  - A. Kinds of positions　肢位の種類 ………………… 2
- **1-2.** Ranges of Motion (ROM)　関節可動域 ………… 3
- **1-3.** Activities　動作 ……………………………………… 4
- **1-4.** Gaits　歩行 …………………………………………… 5

2. Examinations, Findings and Evaluation 検査・測定・評価 ……………………………………… 7

- **2-1.** Examinations　検査・測定 ………………………… 7
  - A. Physical Examinations　身体・運動検査 ……… 7
  - B. Pulmonary Function Tests　肺機能検査 ……… 10
  - C. Eyesight Tests　視力検査 ……………………… 10
  - D. Audiometry　聴力検査 ………………………… 11
  - E. Intelligence Tests　知能関連検査 ……………… 11
  - F. Psychological Tests　心理検査 ………………… 12
- **2-2.** Assessment and Evaluation　評価 ……………… 13

3. Diagnoses and Therapies　診断・治療 ……… 17

- **3-1.** Surgical Treatments　外科的治療 ……………… 18
- **3-2.** Pharmacotheray　薬物療法 ……………………… 19
- **3-3.** Therapies, Trainings and Exercises 療法・作業・訓練・運動 20
  - A. Occupational Therapies　作業療法 …………… 23
  - B. Trainings　訓練 ………………………………… 23
  - C. Exercises and Movements　運動 ……………… 24
  - D. Care　ケア ……………………………………… 25

4. Prostheses and Orthoses　義肢・装具 …………… 26
4-1. Prostheses　義肢 ……………………………………… 26
- A. Structure　構造 …………………………………… 26
- B. Types　種類 ……………………………………… 26
- C. Parts　構成要素 …………………………………… 26

4-2. Upper Limb Prosthesis　義手 ……………………… 27
- A. Types　種類 ……………………………………… 27
- B. Parts Amputated　切断部位による分類 ………… 27
- C. Parts　構成要素 …………………………………… 27

4-3. Lower Limb Prosthesis　義足 ……………………… 28
- A. Types　種類 ……………………………………… 28
- B. Parts　構成要素 …………………………………… 28

4-4. Orthosis　装具 ………………………………………… 29
- A. Materials　材質種類別 …………………………… 29
- B. Upper Limb Orthosis　上肢装具 ………………… 29
- C. Lower Limb Orthosis　下肢装具 ………………… 30
- D. Spinal Orthosis　体幹装具 ………………………… 31
- E. Corsets　コルセット ……………………………… 31
- F. Splints　スプリント（副子）……………………… 31

5. Devices　福祉機器・用具 …………………………………… 32
5-1. Assistive Devices (Equipment)　補助器具 ………… 33
5-2. Medical Treatment Tools　処置用具 ……………… 34

6. Fields, Occupations, Persons and Institutions
リハビリテーションの領域・職種・対象者・制度 …… 35
6-1. Fields　領域 …………………………………………… 35
6-2. Occupations　職種 …………………………………… 35
6-3. Persons　対象者 ……………………………………… 36
6-4. Institutions　制度 …………………………………… 37

7. Facilities and Organizations　施設・組織 …………… 38
7-1. Facilities for Physical Handicaps 肢体不自由者のための施設 … 39

8. Risk Management　リスクマネジメント ············· 41

Part 2　Medical Terms　医学・医療の基本英単語　　43

1. Symptoms and Findings　症状・所見 ············· 44

2. Diseases and Disorders of the Musculoskeletal System
   筋骨格系の疾患・障害 ································ 54
   - 2-1. Bones　骨 ·· 54
   - 2-2. Joints　関節 ····································· 55
   - 2-3. Muscles, Tendons and Ligaments　筋肉・腱・靭帯　58
   - 2-4. Movements and Gaits　運動・歩行 ············· 59

3. Diseases and Disorders of the Circulatory System
   循環系の疾患・障害 ·································· 61
   - 3-1. Heart　心臓 ····································· 61
   - 3-2. Blood Vessels　血管系 ························· 62

4. Diseases and Disorders of the Nervous System
   脳神経系の疾患・障害 ································ 64
   - 4-1. Brain　脳 ·· 64
   - 4-2. Nervous System　神経系 ······················· 66

5. Diseases and Disorders of the Sense Organs and Throat
   感覚器官の疾患・障害 ································ 70
   - 5-1. Eye　眼 ·· 70
   - 5-2. Ear　耳 ·· 72
   - 5-3. Nose and Throat　鼻・咽喉 ···················· 73
   - 5-4. Skin　皮膚 ······································· 74

6. Diseases and Disorders of the Respiratory System
   呼吸器系の疾患・障害 ································ 78

7. **Diseases and Disorders of the Digestive System**
   消化器系の疾患・障害 ……………………… 80
   - **7-1.** Dentistry / Oral Surgery　歯科・口腔外科 ……… 82

8. **Diseases and Disorders of the Genitourinary System**
   腎・尿路系の疾患・障害 …………………… 84

9. **Diseases and Disorders of the Reproductive System**
   生殖系の疾患・障害 ………………………… 87
   - **9-1.** Pregnancy and Childbirth　妊娠・出産 ………… 88

10. **Diseases and Disorders of the Immune System**
    免疫系の疾患・障害 ………………………… 90
    - **10-1.** Systemic Autoimmune Diseases; Collagen Diseases
      全身性自己免疫疾患；膠原病 …………………… 90
    - **10-2.** Immunodeficiency Diseases (Disorders)
      免疫不全症 ……………………………………… 91

11. **Endocrine, Nutritional and Metabolic Diseases**
    内分泌・栄養・代謝疾患 …………………… 92
    - **11-1.** Endocrine Diseases and Disorders
      内分泌疾患・障害 ……………………………… 92
    - **11-2.** Nutritional and Metabolic Diseases and Disorders
      栄養・代謝疾患・障害 ………………………… 94

12. **Hematopoietic Diseases**　造血系疾患 ………… 97

13. **Congenital and Hereditary Diseases and Disorders**
    先天性／遺伝性の疾患・障害 ……………… 101

14. **Mental Health Diseases and Disorders**
    心因性・精神疾患と障害 …………………… 104

15. **Infectious Diseases**　感染症 ………………… 109
    - **15-1.** Pathogenic organisms　病原微生物 ………… 111

Part 3 Terms of Body Parts and Functions
人体各部の名称と機能の英単語   113

1. Head and Neck　頭頚部 ……………………………… 114
- **1-1.** Bones, Ligaments and Joints　骨・靭帯・関節 … 114
- **1-2.** Muscles　筋肉 ……………………………… 115
- **1-3.** Nerves　神経 ……………………………… 117
- **1-4.** Blood Vessels　血管 ……………………………… 118
- **1-5.** Brain　脳 ……………………………… 119
- **1-6.** Ear　耳 ……………………………… 121
- **1-7.** Eye　眼 ……………………………… 122
- **1-8.** Nose　鼻 ……………………………… 122
- **1-9.** Mouth　口 ……………………………… 123
- **1-10.** Skin　皮膚 ……………………………… 123

2. Back and Spinal Cord　背部と脊髄 ……………… 125
- **2-1.** Bones, Ligaments and Joints　骨・靭帯・関節 … 125
- **2-2.** Muscles　筋肉 ……………………………… 126
- **2-3.** Nerves　神経 ……………………………… 127

3. Chest　胸部 ……………………………… 128
- **3-1.** Bones, Ligaments and Joints　骨・靭帯・関節 … 128
- **3-2.** Muscles　筋肉 ……………………………… 128
- **3-3.** Nerves　神経 ……………………………… 129
- **3-4.** Blood Vessels　血管 ……………………………… 129
- **3-5.** Heart　心臓 ……………………………… 130
- **3-6.** Respiratory Organs　呼吸器官 ……………… 131

4. Abdomen and Pelvis　腹部・骨盤部 ……………… 132
- **4-1.** Bones, Ligaments and Joints　骨・靭帯・関節 … 132
- **4-2.** Muscles　筋肉 ……………………………… 132
- **4-3.** Nerves　神経 ……………………………… 133
- **4-4.** Blood Vessels　血管 ……………………………… 133

- **4-5.** Digestive Organs　消化器官 ……………………… 134
- **4-6.** Genitourinary Organs　泌尿生殖器官 …………… 135

5. Upper Extremities　上肢 …………………………… 136
- **5-1.** Bones, Ligaments and Joints　骨・靱帯・関節 … 136
- **5-2.** Muscles　筋肉 ………………………………… 138
- **5-3.** Nerves　神経 …………………………………… 139
- **5-4.** Blood Vessels　血管 …………………………… 140

6. Lower Extremities　下肢 …………………………… 141
- **6-1.** Bones, Ligaments and Joints　骨・靱帯・関節 … 141
- **6-2.** Muscles　筋肉 ………………………………… 143
- **6-3.** Nerves　神経 …………………………………… 145
- **6-4.** Blood Vessels　血管 …………………………… 145

7. Histology　組織学用語 ……………………………… 146
- **7-1.** Blood Cells　血液細胞 ………………………… 146
- **7-2.** Tumors　腫瘍 …………………………………… 146

8. Physiology　生理学用語 …………………………… 147
- **8-1.** Head and Neck　頭頸部 ……………………… 147
- **8-2.** Back and Spinal Cord　背部と脊髄 …………… 148
- **8-3.** Chest　胸部 …………………………………… 148
- **8-4.** Abdomen and Pelvis　腹部・骨盤部 ………… 149
- **8-5.** Upper Extremities　上肢 ……………………… 149
- **8-6.** Reactions, Reflexes and Responses　反応, 反射 … 150
- **8-7.** Physiologically Active Substances
　　　生体分子, 生理活性物質 ……………………… 152

Part 4 Useful Expressions for Rehabilitation
リハビリテーションに役立つ英語表現　　155

1. Activities of Daily Living (ADL)　日常生活動作 …… 156
- **1-1.** Interview　面接 ………………………………………… 156
  - A. First time interview / First session　初回面接 …… 156
  - B. Afterward second session　2回目以降 …………… 157
- **1-2.** Transfer Activities　移乗・移動動作 ……………… 159
- **1-3.** Housework Activities　家事動作 …………………… 161
  - A. Cleaning　掃除 ………………………………………… 161
  - B. Cooking　調理 ………………………………………… 162
  - C. Washing clothes　洗濯 ……………………………… 163
  - D. Shopping　買物 ……………………………………… 163
  - E. Other activities　その他 ……………………………… 164
- **1-4.** Dressing Activities　更衣動作 ……………………… 164
- **1-5.** Feeding Activities　食事動作 ………………………… 166
  - A. Before and after the meal　食前，食後 …………… 168
  - B. Taking medicine　薬の服用 ………………………… 168
- **1-6.** Grooming Activities　整容動作 ……………………… 169
  - A. Hand-washing　手洗い ……………………………… 169
  - B. Face-washing　洗顔 ………………………………… 170
  - C. Tooth-brushing　歯磨き …………………………… 171
  - D. Hair-washing　洗髪 ………………………………… 171
  - E. Cutting nails　爪切り ………………………………… 172
  - F. Shaving / Making up　ひげ剃り/化粧 …………… 172
- **1-7.** Bathing Activities　入浴動作 ………………………… 172
- **1-8.** Toilet Activities　排泄動作 …………………………… 174
- **1-9.** Standard of Exercises for ADL
  日常生活動作のための基本的運動 ………………… 176
  - A. Exercises anywhere　どこでもできる運動 ……… 177
  - B. Basic exercises　基本運動 ………………………… 177

1-10. Basic Training of Techniques for Occupational Therapy
　　　基礎作業療法 ·············· 179
　A. Ceramics　陶芸 ·············· 180

2. Physical Exercises　身体運動 ·············· 182
2-1. Basic Exercises　基本的運動 ·············· 182
2-2. Basic Range of Motion (ROM) Exercise
　　　基本的可動域運動 ·············· 184
　A. Exercise of joints　関節の運動 ·············· 184
　B. Stretching　ストレッチング ·············· 185
　C. Muscle-strengthening exercise　筋力増強運動 ····· 186
　D. Strengthening abdominal muscles　腹筋の強化 ··· 187
　E. Exercise of resistive movement　抵抗運動 ·············· 187
　F. Walking, going up and down stairs, transferring
　　　歩行，階段昇降，移乗 ·············· 188
2-3. Manual Dexterity Exercises of Fingers
　　　手指巧緻性訓練 ·············· 190
　A. Exercises with pegboard　ペグボード訓練 ·············· 190

3. Rehabilitation for Diseases　疾患別リハビリテーション 192
3-1. Diseases of Locomotive Organs　運動器疾患 ······ 192
　A. Fracture　骨折 ·············· 192
　B. Muscular injuries / Tendon injuries
　　　筋損傷 / 腱損傷 ·············· 197
　C. Arthritis　関節炎 ·············· 199
　D. Inversion strain of ankle joint　足関節内反捻挫 ··· 200
　E. Amputation　切断 ·············· 201
　F. Lower back pain　腰痛 ·············· 202
3-2. Cerebrovascular Accidents　脳血管障害 ·············· 204
　A. Activity of turning over　寝がえり動作 ·············· 205
　B. Activity of self-lifting　起き上がり動作 ·············· 206
　C. Activity of standing up　立ち上がり動作 ·············· 206
　D. Walking exercises　歩行練習 ·············· 207

E. Functional training of the upper limb
      上肢機能訓練 …………………………………… 207
   F. Facilitation to the adduction of the hip joint muscle
      股関節内転筋促進 ……………………………… 208
3-3. Chronic Obstructive Pulmonary Disease (COPD)
   慢性閉塞性呼吸器疾患 ……………………………… 208
   A. Abdominal breathing training　腹式呼吸練習 …… 208
   B. Panic control in the sitting position
      座位でのパニックコントロール ………………… 209
3-4. Peripheral Nerve Injury　末梢神経損傷 ………… 209
   A. In the early stage　初期の段階で ……………… 209
   B. ROM (range of motion) exercise of the upper extremity
      上肢可動域訓練 ………………………………… 210
3-5. Parkinson Disease　パーキンソン病 …………… 211
   A. Transferring hoops to other quoits　輪投げの輪移し 211
   B. Sanding movement　サンディング …………… 211
3-6. Spinal Cord Injury　脊髄損傷 …………………… 212
   A. C5 complete spinal cord injury　C5完全脊髄損傷 … 212
   B. Pressure elimination　除圧動作 ……………… 213
   C. Cervical central cord injury　中心性頸髄損傷 …… 214
3-7. Rheumatoid Arthritis　関節リウマチ …………… 215
   A. Active movement of finger joints　手指関節の自動運動 215
   B. Exercise for having a good posture
      作業の間に良い姿勢を保つ運動 ……………… 216
   C. Paraffin bath　パラフィン浴 ………………… 217
3-8. Dysphagia　嚥下障害 …………………………… 218
   A. Warming-up exercise before meal　食前の準備運動 218
   B. Before and during a meal　食前・食事中 ……… 219

日本語索引 …………………………………………… 220
INDEX（英語索引） ………………………………… 244
Abbreviations（略語一覧） ………………………… 271
著者紹介・参考文献 ………………………………… 279

Part 1

Rehabilitation Terms

リハビリテーションの
基本英単語

1. Positions, Ranges of Motion, Activities and Gaits
肢位・体位・姿勢・関節可動域・動作・歩行

1-1. Positions and Postures　　肢位・体位・姿勢

- □ **position** — 肢位, 体位
  - □ anatomical position — 解剖学的肢位
  - □ functional position — 機能的肢位, 良肢位
  - □ fundamental (neutral) position — 基本的肢位
- □ **posture** — 姿勢
  - □ abnormal posture — 異常姿勢

A. Kinds of positions　　肢位の種類

- □ **crouching position** — かがみ肢位
- □ half side-lying position — 半側臥位
- □ half-sitting position — 中腰位
- □ kneeling position — 膝立位
- □ lateral position; side-lying position — 側臥位；横臥位
- □ prone position — 腹臥位
- □ recumbent position; lying position — 臥位
- □ **sitting position** — 座位
  - □ chair sitting position — 椅座位
  - □ crossed leg sitting position — あぐら座位
  - □ Fowler position; semi-sitting position — ファウラー位；半座位
  - □ kneel sitting position — 正座位, 膝座位
  - □ long sitting position — 長座位
- □ **standing position** — 立位
  - □ anterior standing position — 前傾位
  - □ posterior standing position — 後傾位
- □ **supine position; dorsal position** — 仰臥位；背臥位
- □ upright position — 直立位

Part 1 **Rehabilitation Terms** リハビリテーションの基本英単語

1-2. Ranges of Motion (ROM) 関節可動域

- **abduction** 外転《側方への挙上 ⇔ adduction》
  - horizontal abduction 水平外転《肩 = horizontal extension》
  - palmar abduction 掌側外転《母指・手》
  - radial abduction 橈側外転《母指・手》
- **adduction** 内転《⇔ abduction》
  - horizontal adduction; horizontal flexion 水平内転；水平屈曲《肩》
  - palmar adduction 掌側内転《手》
  - ulnar adduction 尺側内転《母指・手》
- **bending** 屈曲《= flexion》
  - lateral bending 側屈《胸・腰部》
  - leftward bending 左屈
  - rightward bending 右屈
- **circumduction** 分回し
  - inward circumduction 内分回し
  - outward circumduction 外分回し
- **depression** 引き下げ，下制，低下
  《肩・顎 ⇔ elevation》
- **deviation** 偏位
  - radial deviation 橈屈《= radial flexion》
  - ulnar deviation 尺屈《= ulnar flexion》
- **elevation** 挙上《⇔ depression》
  - backward elevation 後方挙上《肩》
  - forward elevation 前方挙上《肩》
- **eversion** 外がえし，外反《⇔ inversion》
- **extension** 伸展《⇔ flexion》
  - horizontal extension 水平伸展《肩 = horizontal abduction》
- **flexion** 屈曲《= bending》
  - anteflexion 前屈《頸部・胸腰部》
  - backward flexion 後方挙上《肩》

1	☐ dorsiflexion	背屈《手・頚部・胸腰部》
2	☐ forward flexion	前方挙上《肩》
3	☐ horizontal flexion	水平屈曲《= horizontal adduction》
4	☐ palmar flexion	掌屈《手》
5	☐ plantar flexion	底屈《足・足根》
6	☐ radial flexion	橈屈《手首・手 = radial deviation》
7	☐ ulnar flexion	尺屈《手首・手 = ulnar deviation》
8	☐ **inversion**	**内がえし，内反**《⇔ eversion》
9	☐ **opposition**	**対立**《母指》
10	☐ **pronation**	**回内**《前腕・足 ⇔ supination》
11	☐ **protrusion; protraction**	**前突**《下顎》
12	☐ **retrusion; retraction**	**後退**《下顎》
13	☐ **rotation**	**回旋**《頚部，胸腰部》
14	☐ external rotation	外旋《肩・殿》
15	☐ internal rotation	内旋《肩・殿》
16	☐ leftward rotation	左旋
17	☐ rightward rotation	右旋
18	☐ **supination**	**回外**《前腕・足 ⇔ pronation》

1-3. Activities　　動作

21	☐ **activities of daily living (ADL)**	**日常生活動作**
22	☐ activities parallel to daily living (APDL)	生活関連動作
23	☐ basic activities of daily living (BADL)	基本日常生活動作
24	☐ ambulation activity	歩行動作
25	☐ bathing activity	入浴動作
26	☐ dressing activity	更衣動作
27	☐ feeding activity	食事動作
28	☐ grooming activity	整容動作
29	☐ home making (housework) activity	家事動作
30	☐ locomotion activity	移動動作

Part 1 **Rehabilitation Terms** リハビリテーションの基本英単語

- [ ] stair climbing — 階段昇降
- [ ] toileting — 排泄動作，トイレ動作
- [ ] transfer activity — 移乗動作
- [ ] wheelchair activity — 車椅子動作

1-4. Gaits　歩行

- [ ] bottom hitching — いざり這い
- [ ] bucking — 膝折れ
- [ ] cadence — 歩調
- [ ] cadence rate; walking rate — 歩行率
- [ ] center of gravity — 重心
- [ ] **claudication** — **跛行**
- [ ] intermittent claudication — 間欠性跛行
- [ ] creeping — ずり(肘)這い
- [ ] fall — 転倒
- [ ] foot flat — 足底接地
- [ ] **gait** — **歩行，歩き方，足取り**
- [ ] gait velocity — 歩行速度
- [ ] half kneeling — 片膝立ち
- [ ] hop on one leg — 片足跳び
- [ ] leg discrepancy — 脚長差
- [ ] push off — 踏みきり，プッシュオフ
- [ ] **standing** — **起立**
- [ ] standing on one leg — 片足立ち
- [ ] standing on tiptoe — つま先立ち
- [ ] **step** — **一歩，歩み**
- [ ] step length — 歩長
- [ ] step width — 歩幅(ほほく)
- [ ] **stride** — **重複歩，ストライド**
- [ ] stride length — 重複歩長，ストライド長

5

1	stride width	重複歩幅，ストライド幅
2	**walk [ing]**	**歩行**
3	automatic walking	自動歩行
4	staggering walk	よろめき歩き
5	walk with support	つたい歩き
6	walk without help	ひとり歩き，独歩

COLUMN　医療の場に関わる人々の英語

医療従事者を表すコ・メディカルという呼称が使われ始めて久しい。既に日本の辞書に記載されているものの，これは和製英語である。また，comedic（喜劇的な，こっけいな）という英語があるので，発音，アクセントには要注意である。さて，医療の場に関わる人々の呼び方には語源を知ると興味ぶかいものが多い。(Gk.＝ギリシャ語，以外はラテン語)

- patient(患者)：pathos(Gk. 苦痛，感情) + -ent(行為者)→ 苦しむ人。
- physician(医師，特に内科医)：physis(Gk. 自然) +-ian(…に精通する人)→ 自然科学を応用して医学を実践する人。
- surgeon(外科医)：cheir(Gk. 手)+-on((…に精通する人)
- nurse(看護師)：nutrix(ミルク)を与える人。→ 病の療養を世話し，診療の補助をする人。nutritionist(栄養士)も同源。

そして，physical therapist(理学療法士)，occupational therapist(作業療法士)，speech language-hearing therapist(言語聴覚士)に共通するtherapistは，「therapy(Gk. therapeía: 付き添う・治癒) + -ist(行う人)」を語源とする。そこには，投薬や外科手術によって患者を治療する医師とは異なり，patient(患者)と共にあって援助，治療する意味が含まれていると言える。なるほどザ・職種と納得できよう。

Part 1 **Rehabilitation Terms**　リハビリテーションの基本英単語

2　Examinations, Findings and Evaluation
検査・測定・評価

2-1. Examinations　　　　　　　　　　検査・測定

A. Physical Examinations　　　　　　　身体・運動検査

- [ ] action potential　　　　　　　　　　活動電位
  - [ ] compound motor action potential (CMAP)　複合運動活動電位
  - [ ] compound muscle action potential (CMAP)　複合筋活動電位
- [ ] Behavioural Inattention Test - Japanese version (BIT)　　行動性無視検査
- [ ] Berg Balance Scale (BBS)　　　　　バーグ・バランス尺度
  《バランス機能評価》
- [ ] **blood pressure (BP)**　　　　　　　血圧
  - [ ] basal blood pressure　　　　　　　基礎血圧
- [ ] **checkup**　　　　　　　　　　　　**健康診断**
  - [ ] complete checkup　　　　　　　　精密検査
  - [ ] regular checkup　　　　　　　　　定期健診
  - [ ] thorough medical checkup;
    multiple health screening　　　　　　人間ドック
- [ ] co-ordination test (Cord-T)　　　　　協調性テスト
- [ ] computed tomography (CT)　　　　コンピュータ断層撮影診断〔法〕
- [ ] drink test　　　　　　　　　　　　水飲みテスト
- [ ] electrocardiogram (ECG)　　　　　心電図
- [ ] **electrocardiography (ECG)**　　　　**心電図検査〔法〕**
  - [ ] exercise electrocardiography　　　運動負荷心電図検査
- [ ] electrodiagnosis (EDX)　　　　　　電気診断〔法〕
- [ ] electroencephalogram (EEG);
  brain wave　　　　　　　　　　　　脳波
- [ ] electroencephalography (EEG)　　脳波検査〔法〕
- [ ] electromyogram (EMG)　　　　　　筋電図

1	☐ **electromyography (EMG)**	**筋電図検査〔法〕**
2	☐ finger tapping test	指叩き試験
3	☐ finger to nose to finger test	指鼻指テスト《小脳機能》
4	☐ Functional Independence Measure	機能的自立度評価法
5	(FIM)	
6	☐ grip strength	握力
7	☐ **heart rate (HR)**	**心拍数**
8	☐ **height**	**身長**
9	☐ line bisection test	線分二等分試験
10	☐ magnetic resonance angiography	磁気共鳴血管造影〔法〕
11	(MRA)	
12	☐ magnetic resonance imaging (MRI)	磁気共鳴画像〔法〕
13	☐ manual muscle testing (MMT)	徒手筋力検査法
14	☐ Medical Outcomes Study Short	SF-36健康調査《36項目の質問
15	Form-36 Health Survey (SF-36)	に答える包括的健康関連調査》
16	☐ metabolic rate	代謝率
17	☐ basal metabolic rate (BMR)	基礎代謝率
18	☐ relative metabolic rate (RMR)	エネルギー代謝率
19	☐ motor function test	運動機能テスト
20	☐ myelography	ミエログラフィー，脊椎造
21		影検査
22	☐ nerve conduction velocity (NCV)	神経伝導速度
23	☐ one leg test	片足立ちテスト
24	☐ **positron emission tomography**	**陽電子放出断層撮影〔法〕**
25	**(PET)**	
26	☐ **range of motion test (ROMT)**	**関節可動域テスト**
27	☐ Repetitive Saliva Swallowing Test	反復唾液嚥下テスト
28	(RSST)	
29	☐ Simple Motor Test for Cerebral	脳性麻痺簡易運動検査
30	Palsy (SMTCP)	

Part 1 **Rehabilitation Terms** リハビリテーションの基本英単語

- Simple Test for Evaluating Hand Function (STEF) — 簡易上肢機能テスト
- **single photon emission computed tomography (SPECT)** — **単光子放射断層撮影〔法〕**
- somatosensory evoked potentials (SEPs) — 体性感覚誘発電位
- **sphygmomanometry; blood pressure measurement** — **血圧測定**
- Standard Language Test of Aphasia (SLTA) — 標準失語症検査
- **straight leg raising (SLR) test** — **下肢伸展挙上試験**
- test of activities of daily living — 日常生活動作テスト
- thumb localizing test — 母指探しテスト
- Timed Up and Go (TUG) test — 〔タイムド〕アップアンドゴーテスト《運動機能評価》
- treadmill test (TMT) — トレッドミル試験
- **ultrasonography (US); echography; echo** — **超音波検査〔法〕**；エコー
- vertical suspension test — 垂直吊り下げ試験
- videoendoscopy (VE) — ビデオ内視鏡検査〔法〕
- videofluorography (VF) — ビデオ造影検査〔法〕
- **[body] weight** — **体重**
-   measurement of [body] weight — 体重測定
- Western Aphasia Battery [Test] (WAB; WABT) — ウェスタン失語症統合検査
- Wisconsin Card Sorting Test (WCST) — ウィスコンシンカード分類検査
- work tolerance — 作業耐容性

B. Pulmonary Function Tests 肺機能検査

- [ ] expiratory reserve volume (ERV) — 予備呼気量
- [ ] forced expiratory volume (FEV) — 努力呼気量
- [ ] functional residual capacity (FRC) — 機能的残気量
- [ ] inspiratory capacity (IC) — 最大吸気量, 深吸気量
- [ ] inspiratory reserve volume (IRV) — 予備吸気量
- [ ] **lung compliance** — **肺コンプライアンス**
- [ ] lung volume — 肺気量
- [ ] maximal voluntary ventilation (MVV) — 最大換気量
- [ ] oxygen uptake (VO$_2$) — 酸素摂取(吸収)量
- [ ] pulmonary [viscous] resistance — 肺粘性抵抗
- [ ] residual volume (RV) — 残気量
- [ ] respiratory resistance (Rrs) — 呼吸抵抗
- [ ] spirometer — スピロメーター, 肺活量計
- [ ] tidal volume (VT) — 一回換気量
- [ ] total lung capacity (TLC) — 全肺気量
- [ ] ventilation threshold (VT) — 換気性作業閾値
- [ ] **vital capacity (VC)** — **肺活量**
  - [ ] forced vital capacity (FVC) — 〔努力〕呼気肺活量
  - [ ] percent vital capacity — パーセント(%)肺活量

C. Eyesight Tests 視力検査

- [ ] Developmental Test of Visual Perception (DTVP) — 視覚発達検査
- [ ] examining near visual acuity and adjusting power — 調節力検査
- [ ] eye examination — 検眼
- [ ] funduscopy; fundus examination — 眼底検査

1	☐ ocular dysmetria	眼ディスメトリア；眼球運動測定異常
3	☐ ophthalmometry	角膜曲率測定
4	☐ **optometry**; **eyesight test**	**視力検査**
5	☐ eyesight test chart; eye chart	視力検査表
6	☐ perimetry; campimetry; visual field test	視野検査
7	☐ refractometry; refraction test	屈折検査
8	☐ swinging flashing test	交互対光反応試験
9	☐ therapeutic eye exercises	視力回復運動
10	☐ tonometry	眼圧測定〔法〕
11	☐ visual acuity correction inspection	視力矯正検査
12	☐ visual recognition memory test	視覚認知検査

D. Audiometry 聴力検査

15	☐ acoustic reaction	音響反射
16	☐ **audiometry**	**聴力検査**
17	☐ objective audiometry	他覚的聴力検査
18	☐ pure tone audiometry	純音聴力検査
19	☐ speech audiometry	語音聴力検査
20	☐ bone conduction	骨〔伝〕導
21	☐ intelligibility of speech	語音明瞭度
22	☐ speech audiogram	スピーチオージオグラム
23	☐ speech discrimination score	語音明瞭度検査
24	☐ speech reception threshold	語音聴取閾値
25	☐ tuning fork	音叉

E. Intelligence Tests 知能関連検査

28	☐ Clock Drawing Test (CDT)	時計描画テスト
29	☐ degree of independent living for demented elderly	認知症高齢者の日常生活自立度

1	☐ dementia rating scale	認知症評価尺度
2	☐ Denver Developmental Screening Test, revised Japanese version (JDDST-R)	改訂日本版デンバー式発達スクリーニング検査
5	☐ [Goodenough] Draw-A-Man (DAM) Intelligence Test	グッドイナフ人物画知能検査
7	☐ everyday memory checklist	生活健忘チェックリスト
8	☐ Kaufman Assessment Battery for Children (K-ABC)	カウフマン児童知能検査
10	☐ mini-mental state examination (MMSE)	簡易知能検査
11	☐ Miyake Paired Verbal Associate Learning Test	三宅式記銘力検査
13	☐ Tanaka-Binet Test	田中・ビネー知能検査

F. Psychological Tests —— 心理検査

16	☐ Bender Gestalt Test (BGT); Bender Visual Motor Gestalt Test	ベンダーゲシュタルト検査
18	☐ drawing test	描画テスト
19	☐ House-Tree-Person (HTP) Test	家屋−樹木−人物画法テスト
20	☐ Illinois Test of Psycholinguistic Abilities (ITPA)	イリノイ精神言語能力検査
22	☐ Kohs Block Design Test	コース立方体組合せテスト
23	☐ Minnesota Multiphasic Personality Inventory (MMPI)	ミネソタ多面人格目録
25	☐ operant behavior	オペラント行動
26	☐ Rorschach Test	ロールシャッハテスト
27	☐ Southern California Sensory Integration Tests (SCSIT)	南カリフォルニア感覚統合検査
29	☐ Subjective Well-being Inventory (SUBI)	心の健康自己評価質問紙

Part 1 **Rehabilitation Terms** リハビリテーションの基本英単語

1. ☐ Thematic Apperception Test (TAT) 主題統覚検査
2. ☐ Tower of Hanoi ハノイの塔《パズルゲーム》
3. ☐ two-point discrimination 二点識別覚《乳幼児精神発達診断法》
5. ☐ Uchida-Kraepelin Performance Test 内田－クレペリン精神作業検査
6. ☐ Yatabe-Guilford (Y-G) Test 矢田部－ギルフォード性格検査, Y-Gテスト

2-2. Assessment and Evaluation 評価

- ☐ **assessment** **評価**
- ☐ behavioral assessment 行動評価
- ☐ Behavioural Assessment of the Dysexecutive Syndrome (BADS) 遂行機能障害症候群の行動評価
- ☐ clinical assessment 診療評価
- ☐ Craig Handicap Assessment and Reporting Technique (CHART) クレイグ・ハンディキャップ評価・報告法《脊髄損傷患者のQOL評価に用いる質問票》
- ☐ Mann Assessment of Swallowing Ability (MASA) マン嚥下機能評価尺度
- ☐ Stroke Impairment Assessment Set (SIAS) 脳卒中機能障害評価法
- ☐ **body mass index (BMI)** **体格指数**
- ☐ **classification** **分類**
- ☐ Frankel classification (scale) フランケル分類《脊髄損傷後の神経学的評価法》
- ☐ Gross Motor Function Classification System (GMFCS) 粗大運動機能分類システム
- ☐ International Classification of Functioning, Disability and Health (ICF) 国際生活機能分類《ICIDHの改訂版》

☐	International Classification of Impairments, Disabilities and Handicaps (ICIDH)	国際障害分類
☐	International Standards for Neurological Classification of Spinal Cord Injury (ISNCSCI)	脊髄損傷後の残存自律神経機能の国際評価基準
☐	International Statistical Classification of Diseases and Related Health Problems, 10th edition (ICD-10)	疾病および関連保健問題の国際統計分類第10版
☐	Keith-Wagener classification	キース・ワゲナーの分類《眼底所見に基づく高血圧の進行度》
☐	Revision of Eichner's classification	修正アイヒナー分類《歯の欠損状態による咬頭嵌合位や咬合支持能力の分類》
☐	Scheie classification	シェイエの分類法《眼底所見による高血圧網膜症の分類》
☐	Steinbrocker classification	スタインブロッカー分類《関節リウマチの進行度と機能障害の分類》
☐	2010 ACR-EULAR classification criteria for rheumatoid arthritis	関節リウマチ分類基準《ACR: American College of Rheumatology 米国リウマチ学会, EULAR: European League Against Rheumatism 欧州リウマチ学会議》
☐	**criteria**	**基準**
☐	Hugh-Jones Dyspnea Criteria	ヒュー・ジョーンズ分類《運動時の呼吸困難度の分類》
☐	Revised ARA Criteria for Rheumatoid Arthritis in Japan	修正日本ARAの診断基準
☐	degree of the bedridden	寝たきり度
☐	developmental quotient (DQ)	発達指数
☐	**evaluation**	**評価**
☐	first evaluation	初期評価

Part 1 **Rehabilitation Terms** リハビリテーションの基本英単語

1	☐ **index**	指数
2	☐ Barthel Index (BI)	バーセルインデックス《ADL評価法》
3	☐ Beck Depression Index (BDI)	ベックうつ病指数
4	☐ **intelligence quotient (IQ)**	知能指数
5,6	☐ **metabolic equivalents (METs, MET)**	メッツ，メット《代謝に相当する値＝身体活動の強度：アメリカスポーツ医学会》
7	☐ **method**	方法
8,9	☐ Bobath method	ボバース法《脳性麻痺・脳血管障害の治療概念》
10,11	☐ Vojta method	ボイタ法《乳児の脳性運動障害の早期診断・治療・リハビリ法》
12-15	☐ PULSES Profile (Physical condition, Upper limb function, Lower limb function, Sensory function, Excretory function, Support)	身体状況，上肢機能，下肢機能，感覚機能，排尿・排泄機能プロフィール《支援の評価要素》
16	☐ **quality of life (QOL)**	〔日常〕生活の質
17	☐ **questionnaire**	質問票
18,19	☐ St George's Respiratory Questionnaire (SGRQ)	聖ジョージ〔病院〕呼吸障害質問票
20	☐ reevaluation	再評価
21	☐ residual function	残存機能
22	☐ satisfaction in daily life (SDL)	日常生活満足度
23	☐ **scale**	尺度
24	☐ Activities of Daily Living Scale	日常生活動作評価尺度
25	☐ Glasgow Coma Scale (GCI)	グラスゴー昏睡尺度
26,27	☐ Hasegawa Dementia Scale – Revised (HDS-R)	長谷川式簡易認知症評価スケール改訂版
28,29	☐ Japan Stroke Scale – Higher Cortical Function (JSS-H)	脳卒中高次脳機能障害重症度スケール
30	☐ Japan Stroke Scale – Mortality (JSS-M)	脳卒中運動機能障害重症度スケール

☐	Life Assessment Scale for the Mentally Ill (LASMI)	精神障害者社会生活評価尺度
☐	Positive and Negative Syndrome Scale (PANSS)	陽性・陰性症状評価尺度
☐	Self-Rating Depression Scale (SDS)	自己評価抑うつ尺度
☐	Wechsler Adult Intelligence Scale – Revised (WAIS-R)	ウェクスラー成人知能検査〔評価尺度〕改訂版
☐	Wechsler Memory Scale – Revised (WMS-R)	ウェクスラー記憶検査〔評価尺度〕改訂版
☐	Wechsler Preschool and Primary Scale of Intelligence – Revised (WPPSI-R)	ウェクスラー就学前・小学生知能検査〔評価尺度〕改訂版
☐	**score**	**評点**
☐	intelligence standard score (ISS)	知能偏差値
☐	**sign**	**徴候**
☐	Kernig sign	ケルニッヒ徴候《髄膜炎等の神経学的検査法》
☐	Lasegue sign	ラセーグ徴侯《膝伸展下肢挙上検査 → straight-leg- raising (SLR) test》
☐	Tinel sign	ティネル徴候
☐	**stage**	**ステージ**
☐	Brunnstrom (Brs) stage	ブルンストロームステージ《片麻痺回復過程の評価法》
☐	Hoehn-Yahr stage (score)	ホーエン・ヤール重症度分類《パーキンソン病の臨床的重症度の評価尺度》
☐	swallowing grade	嚥下グレード
☐	**threshold**	**閾値**
☐	anaerobics threshold (AT)	無酸素性作業閾値

3 Diagnoses and Therapies
診断・治療

1	arthrokinematic approach (AKA)	関節運動学的アプローチ
2	**auscultation**	**聴診**
3	**diagnosis**	**診断**［複数形 **diagnoses**］
4	preliminary diagnosis	予診
5	**evidence-based medicine (EBM)**	**証拠に基づいた医療**
6	**[medical] history**	**病歴**
7	family history	家族歴
8	past history	既往歴
9	social history	社会歴
10	surgical history	手術歴
11	**informed consent**	**インフォームド・コンセント**
12	inspection	視診
13	**lifestyle**	**生活習慣**
14-15	recommendations for lifestyle modification	生活習慣指導
16	**life support**	**救命処置**
17-18	advanced life support (ALS)	二次的(高度)救命処置《除細動器等を用いる救急処置》
19	basic life support (BLS)	基本の救命処置
20	**medical interview**	**医療面接，問診**
21	narrative-based medicine (NBM)	物語に基づいた医療
22-23	neuro-developmental [approach] to treatment	神経発達学的治療
24-25	neurophysiological approach	神経生理学的アプローチ《＝固有神経性筋促進法》
26-27	occupational disease; industrial disease	職業病

1	☐ outcome	転帰
2	☐ **palpation**	**触診**
3	☐ percussion	打診
4	☐ **prescription**	**処方**
5	☐ exercise prescription	運動処方
6	☐ **prognosis**	**予後**
7	☐ prognostic	前兆となる
8	☐ remission	寛解
9	☐ therapy program	治療プログラム

3-1. Surgical Treatments　　　外科的治療

12	☐ **amputation**	**切断**
13	☐ above elbow (AE) amputation	上肢(AE)切断
14	☐ above knee (AK) amputation	大腿(AK)切断
15	☐ below elbow (BE) amputation	上腕(BE)切断
16	☐ below knee (BK) amputation	下腿(BK)切断
17	☐ Boyd amputation	ボイド切断
18	☐ forequarter amputation	フォークオーター切断《肩甲胸郭間切断》
20	☐ Kirk amputation	カーク切断
21	☐ Krukenberg amputation	クルーケンベルグ切断
22	☐ lower extremity amputation	下肢切断
23	☐ Pirogoff amputation	ピロゴフ切断
24	☐ Syme amputation	サイム切断
25	☐ upper extremity amputation	上肢切断
26	☐ **arthrodesis**	**関節固定術**
27	☐ arthroplasty	関節形成(置換)術
28	☐ bipolar hip arthroplasty	人工骨頭置換術
29	☐ artificial joint replacement	人工関節置換術
30	☐ disarticulation	関節離断〔術〕

Part 1 **Rehabilitation Terms** リハビリテーションの基本英単語

1. ☐ discography — 椎間板造影術
2. ☐ myodesis — 筋肉固定術
3. ☐ osteosynthesis — 骨接合術
4. ☐ reduction — 整復〔術〕
5. ☐ open reduction — 観血的整復〔術〕
6. ☐ tendon grafting — 腱移植術
7. ☐ tendon transfer — 腱移行術
8. ☐ transplant; implant — 移植片
9. ☐ **transplantation; implantation** — **移植〔術〕**

3-2. Pharmacotherapy 薬物療法

12. ☐ adrenocorticosteroid — 副腎皮質ステロイド薬
13. ☐ analgesic; pain killer; pain reliever — 鎮痛薬
14. ☐ anesthetic — 麻酔薬
15. ☐ anorectic; appetite suppressant; appetite depressant — 食欲抑制薬
17. ☐ antiallergic — 抗アレルギー薬
18. ☐ antianxiety drug; anxiolytic — 抗不安薬
19. ☐ antibiotic — 抗生物質, 抗菌薬
20. ☐ anticoagulant; antithrombotic — 抗凝固薬;抗血栓薬
21. ☐ antidepressive agent; antidepressant — 抗うつ薬
23. ☐ antidiarrheal — 止痢薬, 下痢止め
24. ☐ antidote — 解毒薬
25. ☐ antihistamine — 抗ヒスタミン薬
26. ☐ antihyperlipidemic — 抗高脂血症治療薬
27. ☐ antihypertensive; depressor; pressure pill — 降圧薬
29. ☐ anti-inflammatory drug — 抗炎症薬
30. ☐ nonsteroidal anti-inflammatory drugs (NSAIDs) — 非ステロイド抗炎症薬

1	☐ antipyretic; antifebrile	解熱薬
2	☐ antirheumatic drug	抗リウマチ薬
3	☐ antitussive; cough medicine	鎮咳薬；咳止め
4	☐ aspirin	アスピリン《商標》
5	☐ bronchodilator	気管支拡張薬
6	☐ cold medicine; cold remedy	感冒薬
7	☐ digestant; digestive	消化薬
8	☐ diuretic	利尿薬
9	☐ **drug; medicine; remedy**	**薬；薬剤；治療薬**
10	☐ drug administration guidance	薬剤指導，服薬指導
11	☐ laxative; purgative; cathartic	瀉下薬，便通薬，下剤
12	☐ ear drop	点耳薬
13	☐ eye drop	点眼薬
14	☐ generic drug	ジェネリック医薬品
15	☐ hypnotic; sleeping pill	催眠薬；睡眠薬
16	☐ intestinal regulator; bowel	整腸薬
17	medicine	
18	☐ **medication**	**投薬〔法〕，薬物，薬剤**
19	☐ parenteral nutrition	非経口〔的〕栄養〔補給〕
20	☐ psychotropic	向精神薬
21	☐ sedative; narcotics	鎮静薬；麻酔薬，麻薬
22	☐ thrombolytic	血栓溶解薬
23	☐ tranquilizer	精神安定薬，トランキライザー
24	☐ vasodilator drug	血管拡張（弛緩）薬

3-3. Therapies, Trainings and Exercises　療法・作業・訓練・運動

27	☐ alcohol rehabilitation program (ARP)	アルコール中毒リハプログラム
28	☐ **automated external**	**自動体外式除細動器**
29	**defibrillator (AED)**	

Part 1 **Rehabilitation Terms** リハビリテーションの基本英単語

- **cardiopulmonary resuscitation (CPR)** 心肺蘇生法
- **chemotherapy** 化学療法
- electrical stimulation 電気刺激〔法〕
  - functional electrical stimulation (FES) 機能的電気刺激〔法〕
  - therapeutic electrical stimulation (TES) 治療的電気刺激〔法〕
  - transcutaneous electrical nerve stimulation (TENS) 経皮的電気刺激〔法〕
- habilitation 療育
- hydrotherapy 水治療法
- hyperalimentation 高栄養療法
  - intravenous hyperalimentation (IVH) 経静脈高カロリー輸液
- immunotherapy 免疫療法
- infrared treatment 赤外線療法
- **infusion; drip** 点滴
  - intravenous drip 点滴静注
- **injection** 注射
- injector; syringe 注射器
- inoculation 接種
- microwave diathermy (therapy) マイクロ波療法《極超短波療法》
- **occupational therapy** 作業療法
  - occupational therapy outside the hospital 院外作業療法
  - supportive occupational therapy 支持的作業療法
- percutaneous trans-esophageal gastrotubing (gastrostomy) (PTEG) 経皮経食道胃管挿入術
- **physical therapy; physiotherapy** 理学療法
  - chest physical therapy; lung physiotherapy 肺理学療法
- proprioceptive neuro-muscular facilitation (PNF) technique 固有受容性神経筋促進法
- prosthetic and orthotic treatment 義肢・装具療法

1	☐ **radiotherapy**	**放射線療法**
2	☐ **therapy**	**療法**
3	☐ art therapy	芸術療法
4	☐ cognitive-behavioral therapy;	認知行動療法
5	cognitive behavior therapy	
6	☐ conductive heat therapy	伝導熱療法
7	☐ continuative passive motion (CPM) therapy	持続的多動運動療法
8	☐ deep heating therapy	深部温熱療法
9	☐ functional occupational therapy	機能的作業療法
10	☐ life therapy	生活療法
11	☐ low frequency current therapy	低周波療法
12	☐ mind-body therapy	心身リラクゼーション療法
13	☐ prevocational occupational therapy	職業前作業療法
14	☐ radiant heat therapy	輻射熱療法
15	☐ recreation therapy	レクリエーション療法
16	☐ sandplay therapy	箱庭療法
17	☐ sensory integrative therapy	感覚統合療法
18	(approach)	
19	☐ surface heating therapy	表在性温熱療法
20	☐ thermotherapy	温熱療法
21	☐ traction therapy	牽引療法
22	☐ ultra-low temperature therapy	低温療法
23	☐ ultraviolet therapy	紫外線療法
24	☐ **treatment**	**治療**
25	☐ conservative treatment	保存療法
26	☐ **vaccination**	**予防接種**
27	☐ **vaccine**	**ワクチン**
28	☐ bacillus Calmette-Guérin (BCG)	カルメット-ゲラン菌（BCG）
29	vaccine	ワクチン
30		

Part 1 **Rehabilitation Terms**　リハビリテーションの基本英単語

A. Occupational Therapies　作業療法

- ☐ arranging in parallel crosses　井桁組み《木工》
- ☐ cane work　籐細工
- ☐ ceramics　陶芸
- ☐ cloisonné　七宝焼き
- ☐ crossword puzzle　クロスワードパズル
- ☐ drawing for coloring　塗り絵
- ☐ finger painting　フィンガー・ペインティング
- ☐ forming with coils　紐づくり《陶芸》
- ☐ gardening　園芸
- ☐ knitting　編み物
- ☐ leather works　革細工
- ☐ macramé　マクラメ
- ☐ method of making boxes　箱作り法
- ☐ peg board　ペグボード
- ☐ quilting　刺し子，キルティング
- ☐ sanding　やすり磨き，サンディング
- ☐ stamping　刻印打ち《革細工》
- ☐ weaving activity　織物
- ☐ wood carving　木彫り
- ☐ woodworking; woodwork　木工

B. Trainings　訓練

- ☐ breathing exercise　呼吸訓練
- ☐ co-ordinate exercise　協調性訓練
- ☐ exchange handedness　利き手交換
- ☐ medicine ball　メディシンボール
- ☐ muscle re-education exercise　筋再教育訓練
- ☐ muscle relaxation exercise　筋弛緩訓練
- ☐ muscle strengthening exercise　筋肉増強訓練

1 リハビリテーションの基本英単語

1	☐ postural exercise	姿勢訓練
2	☐ range of motion exercise	関節可動域訓練
3	☐ rod exercise	棒訓練
4	☐ **training**	**訓練**
5	☐ autogenic training	自律訓練法
6	☐ bladder training	排尿訓練
7	☐ functional rehabilitation training	機能回復訓練
8	☐ functional training	機能訓練
9	☐ group training	グループ訓練
10	☐ prosthetic training	義肢装具訓練
11	☐ skill training	スキルトレーニング
12	☐ social skill training (SST)	社会生活技能訓練
13	☐ stump training	断端訓練
14	☐ swallowing training	嚥下訓練
15	☐ training in parallel bar	平均棒訓練
16	☐ vocational training	職業訓練

C. Exercises and Movements　運動

19	☐ anaerobics	無酸素性運動
20	☐ **breathing; respiration**	**呼吸**
21	☐ abdominal breathing (respiration)	腹式呼吸
22	☐ pursed lips breathing	口すぼめ呼吸
23	☐ two-steps breathing	二段呼吸
24	☐ **exercise**	**運動，訓練**《全身を動かすこと》
25	☐ active assistive exercise (movement)	自助介助運動
26	☐ Böhler exercise	ベーラー体操
27	☐ Codman exercise	コッドマン体操
28	☐ exercise for low back pain	腰痛体操
29	☐ Frenkel exercise	フレンケル体操
30	☐ Klapp's creeping exercise	クラップの匍匐(ほふく)運動

Part 1 **Rehabilitation Terms** リハビリテーションの基本英単語

1. ☐ resistance (resistive) exercise — レジスタンス運動，抵抗運動
2. ☐ stretching exercise — ストレッチ運動
3. ☐ **motion** — **運動，動き，動作**《動き方》
4. ☐ **movement** — **運動**《何かを動かすこと》
5. ☐ active movement — 自動運動
6. ☐ passive movement — 他動運動
7. ☐ volitional (voluntary) movement — 随意運動

D. Care　ケア

10. ☐ **bath** — **入浴**
11. ☐ bed bath — 清拭(せいしき)
12. ☐ contrast bath — 温冷交替浴
13. ☐ hot air bath — 熱気浴
14. ☐ paraffin bath — パラフィン浴
15. ☐ partial bath — 部分浴
16. ☐ beating — 叩打法
17. ☐ dressing — ドレッシング
18. ☐ hot pack — ホットパック
19. ☐ kneading — 揉捏法(じゅうねつほう)
20. ☐ manual chest stretching — 徒手胸郭伸張法
21. ☐ **massage** — **マッサージ**
22. ☐ ice massage — 氷マッサージ
23. ☐ postural drainage — 体位排痰法
24. ☐ proprioceptive neuro-muscular facilitation (PNF) technique — 固有受容性神経筋促進法
26. ☐ **rubbing** — **強擦法**
27. ☐ **stroking** — **軽擦法**

4 Prostheses and Orthoses
義肢・装具

4-1. Prostheses 義肢

A. Structure 構造

- ☐ body (internal) powered prosthesis — 体内力源義肢(たいないりきげんぎし)
- ☐ endoskeletal prosthesis — 骨格構造義肢
- ☐ exoskeletal prosthesis — 殻構造義肢(かくこうぞうぎし)
- ☐ external powered prosthesis — 体外力源義肢(たいがいりきげんぎし)

B. Types 種類

- ☐ cosmetic prosthesis — 装飾義肢
- ☐ malleolar prosthesis — 果義肢
- ☐ modular prosthesis — モジュラー義肢
- ☐ permanent prosthesis — 本義肢
- ☐ temporary prosthesis — 仮義肢

C. Parts 構成要素

- ☐ buttress — 支持部, 結合部
- ☐ socket — ソケット
- ☐ diagonal socket — ダイアゴナルソケット
- ☐ Icelandic roll-on silicone socket (ICEROSS) — シリコン製内ソケット
- ☐ plug fit type socket — 差し込み用ソケット
- ☐ quadrilateral socket — 四辺形ソケット
- ☐ suction type socket — 吸着式ソケット
- ☐ soft insert — ソフトインサート《義足用》
- ☐ terminal device — 手先《足部》
- ☐ unit [joint] — 継手〔関節〕

4-2. Upper Limb Prosthesis 義手

A. Structure 構造

Purpose of use 使用目的別
- ☐ Arbeitsarm; work arm 作業用義手
- ☐ body-powered upper limb prosthesis; 能動義手；体内力源義手
  functional upper limb prosthesis
- ☐ cosmetic upper limb prosthesis 装飾用義手
- ☐ temporary upper limb prosthesis 仮義手

Specific types 特殊な義手
- ☐ electric upper limb prosthesis 電動義手
- ☐ hybrid type prosthesis ハイブリッドタイプ義手
- ☐ myoelectric upper limb prosthesis 筋電義手
- ☐ silicon rubber prosthesis シリコン製義手

B. Parts Amputated 切断部位による分類

- ☐ elbow disarticulation prosthesis 肘義手
- ☐ finger prosthesis 手指義手
- ☐ partial hand prosthesis 手部義手，手根中手義手
- ☐ shoulder disarticulation prosthesis 肩義手
- ☐ trans-humeral (above elbow) prosthesis 上腕義手
- ☐ trans-radial (below elbow) prosthesis 前腕義手
- ☐ wrist disarticulation prosthesis 手義手

C. Parts 構成要素

- ☐ control cable system コントロールケーブルシステム
- ☐ elbow joint 肘継手
- ☐ harness ハーネス
- ☐ shoulder joint 肩継手

- [ ] terminal device 手先具
- [ ] wrist joint 手継手

4-3. Lower Limb Prostheses 義足

A. Types 種類

Common artificial foot 一般的義足
- [ ] conventional lower limb prosthesis 常用義足
- [ ] endoskeletal lower limb prosthesis 骨格構造義足
- [ ] hemipelvectomy prosthesis 片側骨盤用義足
- [ ] solid ankle cushion heel (SACH) foot サッチ足部
- [ ] temporary lower limb prosthesis 仮義足

Artificial foot for working 作業用義足
- [ ] above knee prosthesis 大腿義足
- [ ] below-knee prosthesis; 下腿義足
  trans-tibial prosthesis
- [ ] hip prosthesis 股義足
- [ ] hybrid type knee ハイブリッドタイプ膝
- [ ] knee disarticulation prosthesis 膝義足
- [ ] lower limb prosthesis for sport スポーツ用義足
- [ ] malleolar prosthesis 果(足根)義足
- [ ] partial foot prosthesis 足根中足義足
- [ ] toe prosthesis 足指義足

B. Parts 構成要素

- [ ] bent knee prosthesis 膝屈曲義足
- [ ] Klenzack joint クレンザック継手
- [ ] modular prosthesis モジュラー義足
- [ ] pylon prosthesis パイロン義足

Part 1 **Rehabilitation Terms**　リハビリテーションの基本英単語

- [ ] rod klenzack　　　　　　　　　　　棒クレンザック《短下肢装具，足継手》
- [ ] single axis knee　　　　　　　　　　単軸ひざ《継手》
- [ ] suction type above knee prosthesis　　吸着式大腿義足
- [ ] Syme prosthesis　　　　　　　　　　サイム義足

4-4. Orthosis　　装具

- [ ] Denis-Browne orthosis　　　　デニス−ブラウン装具
- [ ] Lorenz apparatus　　　　　　ローレンツ固定装具
- [ ] postural supporting device　　座位保持装具
- [ ] stabilizer　　　　　　　　　　立位保持装具
- [ ] therapeutic orthosis　　　　　治療用装具
- [ ] Toronto hip abduction orthosis　トロント装具

A. Materials　　材質種類別

- [ ] leather molded brace　　革装具
- [ ] metal frame orthosis　　金属枠装具
- [ ] plastic orthosis　　　　　プラスチック装具
- [ ] rigid orthosis　　　　　　硬性装具
- [ ] soft orthosis　　　　　　　軟性装具

B. Upper Limb Orthosis　　上肢装具

- [ ] balanced forearm orthosis (BFO)　平均前腕装具
- [ ] elbow joint　　　　　　　　　　　肘継手
- [ ] elbow orthosis　　　　　　　　　　肘装具
- [ ] finger orthosis　　　　　　　　　　指装具
- [ ] halo brace (orthosis)　　　　　　　ハロー装具《頚椎》
- [ ] hand orthosis　　　　　　　　　　手装具
- [ ] hand dorsal orthosis　　　　　　　手背屈装具
- [ ] long opponens wrist hand orthosis　長対立装具

- ☐ prehension orthosis 把持装具
- ☐ short opponens hand orthosis 短対立装具
- ☐ shoulder orthosis 肩装具

C. Lower Limb Orthoses 下肢装具

- ☐ ankle foot orthosis (AFO); short leg brace (SLB) 短下肢装具
- ☐ Batchelor orthosis バチェラー〔型〕装具
- ☐ extension shoe for leg length discrepancy 補高靴《靴型装具》
- ☐ foot orthosis with lateral corrective wedge 足底装具
- ☐ hip-knee-ankle-foot orthosis (HKAFO) 骨盤帯付き長下肢装具
- ☐ hip orthosis 股装具
- ☐ knee orthosis (KO) 膝装具
- ☐ knee-ankle-foot orthosis (KAFO); long leg brace (LLB) 長下肢装具
- ☐ loose abductor brace ぶかぶか装具
- ☐ metatarsal bar 中足骨バー
- ☐ patellar tendon-bearing (PTB) prosthesis 膝蓋腱荷重式下腿義足, PTB免荷装具
- ☐ prothèse tibiale à emboîtage supracondylien (PTES) 顆上ソケット下腿義足
- ☐ reciprocating gait orthosis (RGO) 交互歩行装具
- ☐ shoe horn brace (SHB) 靴べら式装具
- ☐ shoe orthosis; corrective shoes 靴型装具
- ☐ Thomas weight bearing orthosis トーマス免荷装具

Part 1 **Rehabilitation Terms** リハビリテーションの基本英単語

D. Spinal Orthosis　　　　　　　　　　体幹装具

- □ cervical orthosis　　　　　　　　　　頚椎装具
- □ lumbar orthosis　　　　　　　　　　　腰椎装具
- □ orthosis for scoliosis　　　　　　　　側弯症装具
- □ sacroiliac orthosis　　　　　　　　　　仙腸装具
- □ thoracic orthosis　　　　　　　　　　　胸椎装具
- □ Williams type lumbo-sacral orthosis　〔ウイリアムズ型〕腰仙椎装具

E. Corsets　　　　　　　　　　　　　　　コルセット

- □ canvas corset　　　　　　　　　　　　軟性コルセット
- □ Damen korsett《独》; lumbosacral corset　ダーメンコルセット
- □ frame corset　　　　　　　　　　　　　フレームコルセット
- □ hip supporter　　　　　　　　　　　　ヒップサポーター

F. Splints　　　　　　　　　　　　　　　スプリント（副子）

- □ cock-up splint　　　　　　　　　　　手関節背屈装具
- □ long opponens splint　　　　　　　　長対立スプリント（副子）
- □ night splint　　　　　　　　　　　　　夜間用副子
- □ Oppenheimer splint　　　　　　　　オッペンハイマースプリント（副子）
- □ short opponens splint　　　　　　　短対立スプリント（副子）
- □ Thomas splint　　　　　　　　　　　トーマススプリント（副子）
- □ von Rosen apparatus (splint)　　　　フォンローゼン装具（副子）

《von はドイツ貴族の呼称。ローゼン地方出身の，の意味》

5 Devices
福祉機器・用具

1. **arm sling** — アームスリング《シングルストラップ》
2. **braille** — 〔ブライユ式〕点字法
3. braille writing equipment — 点字用具
4. electric braille writer — 電動点字タイプライター
5. manual braille writer — 手動点字タイプライター
6. **cane; [walking] stick; wand** — 杖
7. adjunctive [walking] stick — 歩行補助杖
8. four-legged cane; quad cane — 四点(四脚)杖
9. multiple pointing stick — 多点杖
10. T cane — T字杖
11. tripped cane — 三脚杖
12. **crutch; walking support** — クラッチ，松葉杖
13. platform crutch — 肘台付杖
14. derotation brace — 減捻装具
15. drop ring lock — ドロップ〔リング〕ロック
16. **ergometer** — エルゴメーター
17. bicycle ergometer — 自転車エルゴメーター
18. heel bumper — 踵バンパー
19. Hubbard tank — ハバードタンク
20. knuckle bender — ナックルベンダー
21. reverse knuckle bender — 逆ナックルベンダー
22. Riemenbugel (RB)《独》; Pavlik harness — リーメンビューゲル；パブリック装具
24. safety knee — 〔安全〕膝継手
25. Silesian band — シレジアバンド
26. soft dressing — ソフトドレッシング
27. stoma — ストーマ

Part 1 **Rehabilitation Terms** リハビリテーションの基本英単語

1. ☐ Swiss lock knee joint — スイスロック式膝継手
2. ☐ toe loop — トウループ
3. ☐ **walker** — **歩行器**
4. ☐ reciprocal walker — 交互歩行器
5. ☐ **wheelchair** — **車椅子**
6. ☐ electric wheelchair — 電動車椅子
7. ☐ reclining wheelchair — リクライニング型車椅子

5-1. Assistive Devices(Equipment) 補助器具

10. ☐ aids for extended reach — 遠隔操作用具
11. ☐ assistant dog — 介助犬
12. ☐ **bathroom; toilet; restroom; lavatory** — **洗面所，トイレ，化粧室**
14. ☐ bed and detachable bed board with powered adjustment — 電動調節ベッド
16. ☐ C-bar — Cバー
17. ☐ commode chair — コモードチェア
18. ☐ cutout cushion — 円座
19. ☐ daily living utensil — 日常生活用具
20. ☐ **diaper; didy** — **おむつ**《didyは幼児語》
21. ☐ Gatch bed — ギャッジ（ギャッチ）ベッド
22. ☐ hand-rail and support rail — 〔歩行保持用〕手すり
23. ☐ **hearing-aid** — **補聴器**
24. ☐ **ladder** — **梯子**
25. ☐ placement ladder — 置き梯子
26. ☐ lap board — はめ込みテーブル
27. ☐ lifting platform — 段差解消機
28. ☐ **reacher; extender without gripping function** — **リーチャー**
30. ☐ self-help device — 自助具

1	☐ stairlift	階段昇降機
2	☐ tactile materials for the floor	点字ブロック
3	☐ telephone coil	テレフォンコイル
4	☐ tilt table	傾斜台
5	☐ urinal; bedpan	しびん
6	☐ urine diverters	採尿器

5-2. Medical Treatment Tools　　処置用具

9	☐ **bandage**	**包帯**
10	☐ 　compression bandage	圧迫包帯
11	☐ corrective brace	矯正器具
12	☐ **plaster; Gips**《独》	**ギプス**
13	☐ plaster splint; Gipsschiene《独》	ギプス副子；ギプスシーネ

COLUMN　rehabilitationとは？

　英語のrehabilitationを語の要素に分けると，re(接頭辞：再び)＋語根(言葉の最小単位)habilis(ラテン語：適した)← ability(能力)＋語尾 -ate(～する)＋ -tion(名詞語尾：こと)となる。そこから，「障害を持つ人に対し機能回復訓練を施し，'社会復帰' させること」を表すようになった。

　歴史的には，ヨーロッパをはじめとする世界各地で19世紀後半に肢体不自由児施設が設立され，機能訓練を開始したことが始まりといわれ，アメリカで，第1次・第2次世界大戦で負傷した兵士を社会復帰させるためにリハビリテーションの必要性が強く認識され，専門医，専門職の養成がなされ，制度も発足した。さらに，1980年の国際障害分類(ICIDH)の提唱は，リハビリテーションの発展に大きく寄与している。

　語の説明はこのように短くてすむが，実際の場面でのリハビリテーションは，療法士(therapists)と患者(patients)ともに，気の長い根気(patience)が，時には長期にわたる忍耐(endurance)が求められるであろう。

6. Fields, Occupations, Persons and Institutions
リハビリテーションの領域・職種・対象者・制度

6-1. Fields　　　　　　　　　　　　　領域

- physical medicine　　　　　　　　　物理療法医学，物療医学
- **rehabilitation (REHAB)**　　　　　リハビリテーション
-   acute phase rehabilitation　　　　急性期リハビリテーション
-   cardiac rehabilitation　　　　　　心臓リハビリテーション
-   cognitive rehabilitation　　　　　認知リハビリテーション
-   educational rehabilitation　　　　教育的リハビリテーション
-   holistic rehabilitation　　　　　　包括的リハビリテーション
-   medical rehabilitation　　　　　　医学的リハビリテーション
-   psychiatric rehabilitation　　　　精神医学的リハビリテーション
-   pulmonary rehabilitation　　　　　呼吸リハビリテーション
-   recovery rehabilitation　　　　　　回復期リハビリテーション
-   rehabilitation engineering　　　　リハビリテーション工学
-   social rehabilitation　　　　　　　社会リハビリテーション
-   vocational rehabilitation　　　　　職業的リハビリテーション
- terminal care　　　　　　　　　　　ターミナルケア，終末期医療

6-2. Occupations　　　　　　　　　　職種

- **care manager**　　　　　　　　　　ケアマネジャー
- **care worker**　　　　　　　　　　　介護福祉士
- **case worker**　　　　　　　　　　　ケースワーカー
- **clinical psychologist**　　　　　　臨床心理士
- **home helper**　　　　　　　　　　　ホームヘルパー
- **occupational therapist (OT)**　　作業療法士
- **orthoptist**　　　　　　　　　　　　視能訓練士
- **physical therapist (PT)**　　　　　理学療法士
- **prosthetist and orthotist (PO)**　義肢・装具士

- ☐ **rehabilitation doctor** リハビリテーション医
- ☐ **social worker** ソーシャルワーカー
- ☐ certified social worker 社会福祉士
- ☐ medical social worker (MSW) 医療ソーシャルワーカー
- ☐ psychiatric social worker (PSW) 精神保健福祉士
- ☐ **speech-language-hearing therapist (ST)** 言語聴覚士

6-3. Persons 対象者

- ☐ person (child) with a disability; disabled person (child) 身体障害者(児)
- ☐ person (child) with intellectual and physical disabilities 心身障害者(児)
- ☐ person (child) with intellectual disabilities 知的障害者(児)
- ☐ person (child) with multiple disabilities 重複障害者(児)
- ☐ person (child) with orthopedic impairment 肢体不自由者(児)
- ☐ person (child) with severe intellectual and physical disabilities 重症心身障害者(児)《個人を指す場合はperson, student, child等．総称の場合はpeople, children等を用いる。また最近ではthe disabledやthe handicappedは差別的表現として避けられる傾向にある。》

6-4. Institutions 制度

- [ ] ambulatory rehabilitation (day care) —— 通所リハビリテーション（デイケア）
- [ ] care management —— ケアマネジメント
- [ ] case management —— ケースマネジメント
- [ ] case work —— ケースワーク
- [ ] community rehabilitation —— 地域リハビリテーション
- [ ] commuting care —— 日帰り介護
- [ ] commuting rehabilitation service —— 通所リハビリテーションサービス
- [ ] Employees' Pension Fund (EPF) —— 厚生年金制度
- [ ] High-cost Medical Care Benefits —— 高額療養費支給制度
- [ ] home rehabilitation —— 在宅リハビリテーション
- [ ] in-home care —— 在宅ケア
- [ ] in-home [welfare] services —— 在宅〔福祉〕サービス
- [ ] Law for the Welfare of Physically Disabled Persons —— 身体障害者福祉法
- [ ] medical social work —— 医療社会事業
- [ ] national health insurance —— 国民健康保険
- [ ] physical disability certificate —— 身体障害者手帳
- [ ] primary nursing care requirement authorization —— 要介護認定
- [ ] rehabilitation counseling —— リハビリテーションカウンセリング
- [ ] rehabilitation service —— 機能回復訓練事業
- [ ] short stay —— ショートステイ
- [ ] social hospitalization —— 社会的入院
- [ ] social work —— ソーシャルワーク
- [ ] visiting nursing —— 訪問看護
- [ ] visiting rehabilitation —— 訪問リハビリテーション

7 Facilities and Organizations
施設・組織

1. ☐ day-care center for children with mental retardation — 知的障害児通園施設
2. ☐ **emergency room (ER)** — **救急処置室**
3. ☐ facility for mentally-handicapped persons — 知的障害者のための施設
4. ☐ **hospice** — **ホスピス**
5. ☐ **hospital** — **病院**
6. ☐ acute hospital — 急性期病院
7. ☐ special functioning hospital — 特定機能病院
8. ☐ institution for severely retarded children — 重症遅進児施設
9. ☐ International Organization for Standardization (ISO) — 国際標準化機構
10. ☐ mental welfare center — 精神保健福祉センター
11. ☐ non-governmental organization (NGO) — 非政府組織
12. ☐ non-profit (not-for-profit) organization (NPO) — 非営利組織
13. ☐ official development assistance (ODA) — 政府開発援助
14. ☐ rehabilitation facility for people with mental retardation — 知的障害者更生施設
15. ☐ rehabilitation institutes — リハビリテーション関連施設
16. ☐ sanatorium type sickbed — 療養型病床群
17. ☐ sanatorium type ward — 療養型病棟
18. ☐ **ward** — **病棟**

7-1. Facilities for Physical Handicaps　肢体不自由者のための施設

- ☐ business skill development school for handicapped people　障害者職業能力開発校
- ☐ care house　ケアハウス
- ☐ [in-home] care support center for the elderly　〔在宅〕介護支援センター
- ☐ child guidance center; consultation office for children　児童相談所
- ☐ child rearing facility　保育施設
- ☐ child welfare institution　児童福祉施設
- ☐ community activity support center　共同作業所，地域活動支援センター
- ☐ day-care center　デイケアセンター；昼間保育所
- ☐ economical nursing home for the elderly　介護利用型軽費老人ホーム
- ☐ facility for blind children　盲児施設
- ☐ facility for blind or deaf children　盲・ろう児施設
- ☐ facility for children with mental retardation　知的障害児童施設
- ☐ facility for deaf children　ろう児施設
- ☐ facility of health care services for the elderly　介護老人保健施設
- ☐ group home　グループホーム
- ☐ hospital home for physically handicapped children　肢体不自由児施設
- ☐ long-term care health facility　介護老人福祉施設
- ☐ long-term care insurance facility　介護保険施設
- ☐ multipurpose senior center　高齢者生活福祉センター
- ☐ nursery school　保育所
- ☐ old-age home with moderate fee　軽費老人ホーム

1	☐ private residential home	有料老人ホーム
2	☐ public health center	保健所
3	☐ rehabilitation counseling center	身体障害者更生相談所
4	for physically disabled person	
5	☐ rehabilitation facilities for the	視覚障害者更生施設
6	visually impaired persons	
7	☐ long-term care sanatorium	介護療養型医療施設
8	☐ school for the deaf	ろう学校
9	☐ school for the intellectually disabled,	養護学校
10	the physically disabled and the	
11	health impaired	
12	☐ sheltered workshop for severely	重度身体障害者保護作業所
13	physically handicapped	
14	☐ single parent support facility	母子生活支援施設
15	☐ social insurance office	福祉保健事務所
16	☐ social welfare office	福祉事務所
17	☐ special elderly nursing home	特別養護老人ホーム
18	☐ vocational facility	授産所（施設）
19	☐ welfare center for the elderly	老人福祉センター

8 Risk Management
リスクマネジメント

accountability	アカウンタビリティー，〔説明報告〕責任
adverse drug events	薬剤事故，薬物有害事象
bias	先入観，偏見，バイアス
communication	**コミュニケーション，意志疎通**
continuous quality improvement (CQI)	継続的質の向上，改善
crisis management	〔政治的・社会的〕重大事態の管理，危機管理
critical path; clinical path	**クリティカルパス；クリニカルパス**
diffusion of responsibility	責任の分散
disclosure	〔情報〕開示
fail-safe	フェイルセーフの
fault-tolerance	フォールトトレランス
feedback	フィードバック
high risk person	ハイリスクパーソン《繰り返し間違いをする人》
human error	人為的エラー，人間がおかす間違い
incident report; near-miss or close-call incident	インシデントレポート；ヒヤリハット報告
latent errors	潜在的エラー
malpractice	医療過誤
medical record review (audit)	診療記録の監査
medical representative (MR)	医療(医薬)情報担当者
medical negligence	医療過失
priority	プライオリティー，優先順位

1	☐ protocol	プロトコール，手順書，
2		計画書
3	☐ quality assurance	〔医療の〕質的保証
4	☐ **risk management**	**リスクマネジメント，**
5		**危機管理，医療安全管理**
6	☐ schema	スキーマ，シェーマ
7	☐ second opinion	セカンドオピニオン
8	☐ transparency	透明性
9	☐ wrong-site surgery	部位誤認手術

Part 2

Medical Terms

医学・医療の基本英単語

1 Symptoms and Findings
症状・所見

A

- abuse / 乱用，虐待
- drug abuse / 薬物乱用
- acidosis / アシドーシス
- acquired / 後天性の
- **acute** / **急性の**
- addiction / 中毒，嗜癖（しへき）
- alcoholism / アルコール依存〔症〕
- alkalosis / アルカローシス
- **allergy**; allergic / **アレルギー；アレルギー性の**
- drug allergy / 薬物アレルギー
- food allergy / 食物アレルギー
- anorexia / 食欲不振
- **anxiety** / **不安**
- ascites / 腹水
- atresia / 閉鎖〔症〕
- atrophy / 萎縮
- **attack; seizure; fit** / **発作**
- drop attack; astatic seizure / 転倒発作；失立発作
- heart attack / 心臓発作
- autoimmune / 自己免疫性の

B

- bed-wetting; nocturnal enuresis / おねしょ；夜尿〔症〕
- belch; burp; eructation / げっぷ，おくび
- **benign** / **良性の**
- bilirubinuria / ビリルビン尿

1	☐ bloat; bloating	膨満感
2	☐ blood loss	失血
3	**bruise**	**挫傷**
4	☐ burning sensation	灼熱感

C

7	☐ calcification	石灰沈着
8	☐ chills	悪寒
9	**chronic**; long-standing	**慢性の**
10	☐ clawhand	鷲手
11	☐ cold sweat	冷や汗
12	☐ colic; paroxysm of bellyache	疝痛；腹部の痙攣痛
13	☐ infantile colic	乳児疝痛
14	**coma**	**昏睡**
15	**[common] cold**	**感冒，かぜ**
16	**complaint**	**病訴**
17	☐ chief complaint	主訴
18	**complication**	**合併症**
19	☐ confusion	混乱
20	☐ congenital	先天性の
21	☐ consciousness clouding	意識混濁
22	**contracture**	**拘縮（こうしゅく），固縮**
23	☐ convulsion; seizure; fit	痙攣
24	**cough**	**咳**
25	☐ crackle	断続性ラ音《パチパチ音》
26	☐ coarse crackle	水泡音
27	☐ fine crackle	捻髪音
28	☐ crepitus; crepitation	捻髪音《聴診音》
29	☐ cyanosis	チアノーゼ

D

- **deficiency** — 欠損〔症〕, 欠乏〔症〕
- **deformity** — 変形
  - thoracic deformity — 胸郭変形
- **degeneration** — 変性〔症〕
- **dehydration** — 脱水症
- deprivation — 剥奪, 遮断
  - emotional deprivation — 情動剥奪
  - sensory deprivation — 感覚遮断
  - sleep deprivation — 睡眠剥奪
- **dependence** — 依存〔症〕
  - physical dependence — 身体的依存
- derangement — 障害《機能の乱れ》
- diffuse — びまん(瀰漫)性の
- dilatation — 拡張
- **disability** — 障害《能力の障害, 身体障害》
- **disabled** — 身体障害の
- discharge — 分泌物
- **discomfort** — 不快感
  - epigastric discomfort — 心窩部不快感
- **disease** — 病気, 疾患
- disinhibition — 脱抑制
- **disorder** — 障害《病気等による不調》
  - language disorder — 言語障害
  - mental disorder — 精神障害
  - sleep (sleeping) disorder — 睡眠障害
  - thought disorder — 思考障害
- disorientation — 失見当識, 見当識障害
- **disturbance** — 障害《機能が阻害されること》
  - disturbance in visual field — 視野障害

1	☐ disturbance of consciousness	意識障害
2	☐ disturbance of memory	記憶障害
3	☐ dysfunction	機能不全，機能障害
4	☐ dystrophy	ジストロフィー，形成異常〔症〕

E

7	☐ ecstasy	精神的高揚
8	☐ **edema**; swelling; dropsy	**水腫**；腫脹，腫れ，むくみ
9	☐ effusion	滲出
10	☐ pleural effusion	胸水
11	☐ embolus; *pl.* emboli	塞栓
12	☐ emotional lability	情動不安定
13	☐ epidemic	伝染性の，流行性の
14	☐ **essential**	**本態性の，必須の**

F

17	☐ face flush	顔面紅潮
18	☐ failure	不全
19	☐ faint; syncope	気絶；失神
20	☐ faintness	脱力〔感〕
21	☐ familial	家族性の
22	☐ **fatigue**	**疲労感，倦怠感**
23	☐ **fever**	**発熱**
24	☐ high fever	高熱
25	☐ low grade fever	微熱
26	☐ **finding**	**所見**
27	☐ fissure	裂〔溝〕
28	☐ **foreign body**	**異物**
29	☐ foreign body sensation	異物感
30	☐ fulminant; fulminating	劇症性の

G

- [ ] gangrene — 壊疽
- [ ] general malaise — 全身倦怠感
- [ ] gouty tophus — 痛風結節
- [ ] **growth** — **成長，増殖，腫瘍**

H

- [ ] **handicap** — **障害**《社会的不利益につながる障害》
- [ ] **headache**; cephalalgia — **頭痛**
- [ ] heartburn; pyrosis — 胸やけ
- [ ] hematemesis — 吐血
- [ ] **hemorrhage; bleeding** — **出血**
  - [ ] profuse hemorrhage; massive bleeding — 大量出血
  - [ ] subcutaneous hemorrhage (bleeding) — 皮下出血
- [ ] hereditary — 遺伝性の
- [ ] hiccup — しゃっくり
- [ ] hoarseness — 嗄(さ)声
- [ ] hyperemia — 充血
- [ ] hyperpathia — ヒペルパチー，痛覚過敏
- [ ] hyperthermia — 高体温症
- [ ] hypertrophy — 肥大
  - [ ] adenoid (adenoidal) hypertrophy — アデノイド肥大
- [ ] hypoglycemia — 低血糖症
- [ ] hypothermia — 低体温症

I

- [ ] idiopathic — 特発性の
- [ ] **illness**; ailment — **〔軽い〕病気**
- [ ] impairment — 障害《機能の障害》
  - [ ] trunk impairment — 体幹失調

Part 2 **Medical Terms** 医学・医療の基本英単語

1	☐ **incontinence**	失禁,失調〔症〕
2	☐ affective incontinence	情動失禁
3	☐ **infant**; infantile	乳児,小児;小児(乳児)〔性〕の
4	☐ infarct; infarction	梗塞;梗塞〔症〕
5	☐ **infection**; infectious; infective	感染;感染性の
6	☐ **inflammation**; inflammatory	炎症;炎症性の
7	☐ intermittent	間欠性の
8	☐ itchiness; itching; pruritus	痒み;瘙痒〔症〕

J

11	☐ **jaundice**	黄疸
12	☐ juvenile	青年の,若年〔性〕の

L

15	☐ lightheadedness	頭部ふらふら感
16	☐ lump	しこり
17	☐ lymphopenia	リンパ球減少

M

20	☐ **malignant**	悪性の
21	☐ mucosa; mucosal	粘膜;粘膜の
22	☐ mucus; mucous	粘液;粘液〔性〕の
23	☐ murmur	雑音《聴診音》
24	☐ pulmonary murmur	肺性雑音

N

27	☐ **nausea**	嘔吐感,吐き気,悪心
28	☐ **necrosis**	壊死
29	☐ neonate; neonatal	新生児;新生児〔性〕の
30	☐ night sweat	寝汗,盗汗

☐	**numbness**	しびれ〔感〕

O

- ☐ occult blood — 潜血
- ☐ odynophagia — 嚥下痛(えんげつう)
- ☐ oppressing feeling — 重圧感

P

- ☐ **pain; ache** — **疼痛**
  - ☐ burning pain; causalgia — 灼熱痛；カウザルギー
  - ☐ localized pain — 限局的な痛み
  - ☐ neuropathic pain — 神経原性疼痛
  - ☐ phantom limb pain — 幻肢痛
  - ☐ radiating pain — 放散痛
  - ☐ severe pain — 激痛
  - ☐ stump pain — 断端痛
- ☐ **palpitation** — **動悸**
- ☐ perseverative tendency — 固執傾向
- ☐ perspiration; sweating — 発汗
- ☐ plaque — 斑
  - ☐ pleural plaque — 胸膜斑 (プラーク)
- ☐ **poisoning** — **中毒**
  - ☐ food poisoning — 食中毒
- ☐ **polyp** — **ポリープ**
- ☐ polyposia — 多飲
- ☐ primary — 一次性の，原発性の
- ☐ projection — 投影

R

- □ rale … ラ音《呼吸音 = crackle》
- □ dry rale … 乾性ラ音
- □ moist rale … 湿性ラ音
- □ rebound phenomenon … 反跳現象
- □ **relaxation** … **弛緩**
- □ **remission** … **寛解**
- □ rhinorrhea … 鼻漏,鼻水
- □ rhonchus; *pl.* rhonchi … ラ音,いびき音,類鼾音
- 《呼吸音；低音性の連続性ラ音》
- □ rigidity … 硬直,固縮

S

- □ sausage-like fingers … ソーセージ状指
- □ scar … 瘢痕
- □ **sclerosis** … **硬結**《硬いしこり》
- □ secondary … 二次性の,続発性の
- □ semicoma … 半昏睡
- □ senile … 老年〔性〕の
- □ sneezing; sternutaion … くしゃみ
- □ snore … いびき〔をかく〕
- □ somnolence; drowsiness … 傾眠；眠気
- □ sore … びらん,ただれ
- □ sore throat … 咽喉炎,咽頭炎
- □ **spasm** … **攣縮（れんしゅく）**
- □ spasticity … 痙縮
- □ spoon nail … 匙状爪
- □ **sputum; phlegm** … **喀痰,痰**
- □ bloody sputum … 血痰（けったん）
- □ stenosis … 狭窄〔症〕

☐	stereognosis	立体認知
☐	strawberry tongue	いちご状舌
☐	stupor	昏迷
☐	stuttering; stammering; dysphemia	どもり；構音障害
☐	sunburn	日焼け《ヒリヒリ痛む場合》
☐	suntan	日焼け《きれいに焼けた場合》
☐	suspended animation	仮死
☐	swollen tonsils	扁桃肥大
☐	**symptom**	**症状**
☐	syncope	失神

T

☐	tardive	遅発性の，晩発性の
☐	tenderness	圧痛
☐	thalamic hand	視床手
☐	thrombus	血栓
☐	transient	一過性の
☐	twist; snap; jerk	急な痙攣，痙動

U

☐	**ulcer**	**潰瘍**
☐	undernutrition	低栄養
☐	urinate; make water; piss	排尿する；おしっこする

V

☐	velar sound	〔軟〕口蓋音
☐	**vertigo; dizziness**	**めまい（眩暈）**
☐	**vomiting**; emesis	**嘔吐**

W

- [ ] wandering; walking　　　　　徘徊
- [ ] weakness　　　　　　　　　　脱力感
- [ ] weight loss　　　　　　　　　体重減少
- [ ] weight reduction　　　　　　　痩身化
- [ ] wheezes　　　　　　　　　　喘鳴；笛声音《呼吸音；高音
　　　　　　　　　　　　　　　　性の連続性ラ音》

Y

- [ ] yawn; gape; oscitation　　　　あくび

COLUMN　symptom(症状)とsign(徴候)の違いは？

　病気の診断の拠り所は，患者が経験する不快感，いつもとは異なる痛み・苦痛のような自覚症状(symptom)である。もう一つは，医師が観察し見つける何らかの異常，つまり他覚症状である徴候(sign)である。

　symptom(sym(ギリシャ語：共に)+ -ptom(災いがふりかかる))は，患者自身が何らかの症状を自覚し，訴えることで適切な診断を受け，病気という災いからいち早く抜け出すことができる，と示唆しているようだ。

　しかしながら，世界一の長寿社会にあって健康な日々を過ごすには，例えば，生活習慣病(lifestyle-related illness)の症状を自覚する前に，自らの健康管理(health care)が何よりも大切，と言えそうである。

2 Diseases and Disorders of the Musculoskeletal System 筋骨格系の疾患・障害

2-1. Bones 骨

- achondroplasia — 軟骨形成不全症
- back pain; lumbago — 腰痛，背部痛
- low back pain — 腰痛
- cervical canal stenosis — 頚部脊中管狭窄症
- **fracture (Frx)** — **骨折**
  - Bennet fracture — ベネット骨折
  - Colles fracture — コーレス骨折
  - complex fracture — 複雑骨折
  - compound fracture; open fracture — 開放骨折
  - compression fracture — 圧迫骨折
  - depressed fracture — 陥没骨折
  - fatigue fracture; stress fracture — 疲労骨折
  - femoral neck fracture; fractured neck of femur — 大腿骨頚部骨折
  - fissured fracture; linear fracture — 亀裂骨折
  - fumeral fracture — 上腕骨骨折
  - green stick fracture — 若木骨折
  - Monteggia fracture — モンテギア骨折
  - radial fracture — 橈骨骨折
  - simple fracture; closed fracture — 単純骨折；閉鎖骨折
- gibbus — 突背，角状脊柱後弯
- herniated disc; [intervertebral] disc herniation — 脱出椎間板；椎間板ヘルニア
- humpback, hunchback; kyphosis — 猫背，亀背(きはい)；〔脊柱〕後弯〔症〕
- lordosis — 〔脊柱〕前弯〔症〕

☐ **osteitis**		骨炎
☐ osteitis deformans; Paget disease		変形性骨炎；パジェット病
☐ osteogenesis imperfecta		骨形成不全症
☐ osteomalacia		骨軟化症
☐ **osteoporosis (OP)**		**骨粗鬆（しょう）症**
☐ **osteosarcoma**		**骨肉腫**
☐ overtraining syndrome		オーバートレーニング症候群
☐ scoliosis		〔脊柱〕側弯〔症〕
☐ shoulder-hand syndrome		肩手症候群
☐ spinal [canal] stenosis		脊柱狭窄症
☐ **spondylitis**		**脊椎炎**
☐ ankylosing spondylitis (AS); Marie-Strümpell disease		強直性脊椎炎；マリーーシュトゥリュンペル病
☐ spondylitis deformans		変形性脊椎炎
☐ spondylolisthesis		脊柱すべり症
☐ spondylolysis		脊椎分離〔症〕
☐ spondylosis		脊椎症
☐ strained back; lumbosacral strain		ぎっくり腰，腰仙部挫傷
☐ systemic bone disease		骨系統疾患，全身性骨疾患
☐ torticollis; wryneck		斜頚
☐ traumatic cervical syndrome		外傷後頚部症候群《頚部挫傷，頚椎捻挫》
☐ vertebral-spinal cord tumor		脊柱・骨髄腫瘍

2-2. Joints 関節

☐ achillobursitis		アキレス腱滑液包炎
☐ ankylosis		〔関節〕強直〔症〕
☐ arthralgia		関節痛
☐ **arthritis**		**関節炎**
☐ psoriatic arthritis		乾癬性関節炎

1	☐ articular (joint) contracture	関節拘縮（こうしゅく）
2	☐ articular deformity	関節変形
3	☐ baseball elbow	野球肘
4	☐ bursitis	滑液包炎
5	☐ Charcot joint	シャルコー関節
6	☐ CREST syndrome	CREST 症候群《Calcinosis石灰沈着症; Raynaud phenomenonレイノー現象; Esophageal dysfunction食道蠕動運動低下; Sclerodactyly手指硬化; Telangiectasia毛細血管拡張症》
11	☐ disarticulation; exarticulation	関節離断
12	☐ discoid meniscus	円板状半月，円板状メニスクス
13	☐ **dislocation**; luxation	**脱臼**
14	☐ congenital dislocation of hip joint	先天性股関節脱臼
15	☐ pathologic dislocation	病的脱臼
16	☐ shoulder dislocation	肩関節脱臼
17	☐ drop foot; footdrop	下垂足
18	☐ genu varum; **bowleg**	内反膝；O 脚
19	☐ genu valgum; **knock-knee**	外反膝；X 脚
20	☐ jumper's knee	ジャンパー膝
21	☐ neck-shoulder-arm syndrome	頸肩腕症候群
22	☐ **osteoarthritis (OA)**; osteoarthropathy; arthrosis	**変形性関節症**
24	☐ patellar clonus	膝クローヌス
25	☐ reflex sympathetic dystrophy (RSD)	反射性交感神経性ジストロフィー
27	☐ **rheumatism**	**リウマチ**
28	☐ palindromic rheumatism	回帰性リウマチ

1	**rheumatoid arthritis (RA)**	関節リウマチ
2	juvenile rheumatoid arthritis (JRA)	若年性関節リウマチ
3	malignant rheumatoid arthritis (MRA)	悪性関節リウマチ
4	palindromic rheumatoid arthritis	回帰性関節リウマチ
5	SAPHO syndrome	SAPHO症候群《Synovitis滑膜炎;
6		Acne痤瘡; Pustulosis膿疱症;
7		Hyperostosis骨化過剰症; Osteitis骨炎》
8	scapulohumeral periarthritis;	肩関節周囲炎；五十肩
9	periarthritis scapula-humeralis;	
10	frozen shoulder	
11	spinal deformity	脊柱変形
12	**sprain**	**捻挫**
13	subluxation	亜脱臼
14	**talipes**	**弯足**
15	talipes calcaneus; pes calcaneus	踵足
16	talipes cavus; pes cavus; claw foot	凹足
17	talipes equinovalgus;	外反尖足
18	pes equinovalgus	
19	talipes equinovarus; pes equinovarus;	内反尖足；内反足
20	clubfoot	
21	talipes equinus; pes equinus;	尖足
22	equinus foot	
23	talipes planovalgus	外反扁平足
24	talipes planus; pes planus; flatfoot	扁平足
25	talipes valgus; pes valgus	外反足
26	talipes varus; pes varus	内反足
27	temporomandibular disorders (TMD)	顎関節症
28	tennis elbow	テニス肘
29	ulnar tunnel syndrome	尺骨神経管症候群

2-3. Muscles, Tendons and Ligaments　筋肉・腱・靭帯

- **contracture** — 拘縮（こうしゅく）
  - Volkmann ischemic contracture — フォルクマン虚血性拘縮
- dystonia — 失調〔症〕，ジストニー
  - dystonia musculorum deformans — 変形性筋失調〔症〕
  - torsion dystonia — 捻転性（ねじれ）失調〔症〕
- **ganglion** — ガングリオン
- hamstring muscle injury — ハムストリング損傷
- **muscle weakness** — 筋力低下
- **muscular atrophy** — 筋萎縮〔症〕
  - spinal muscular atrophy — 脊髄性筋萎縮症
  - spinal progressive muscular atrophy — 脊髄進行性筋萎縮症
- **muscular dystrophy** — 筋ジストロフィー
  - congenital muscular dystrophy (CMR) — 先天性筋ジストロフィー
  - Duchenne muscular dystrophy (DMD) — デュシェーヌ型筋ジストロフィー
  - facio-scapulo-humeral muscular dystrophy — 顔面肩甲上腕筋ジストロフィー
  - limb-girdle muscular dystrophy — 肢帯型筋ジストロフィー
  - progressive muscular dystrophy (PMD) — 進行性筋ジストロフィー
- **muscular stiffness** — 筋硬直
- myasthenia — 筋無力症
- **myasthenia gravis (MG)** — 重症筋無力症
- myasthenic syndrome — 筋無力〔症〕症候群
- myotonic dystrophy — 筋緊張性ジストロフィー
- **ossification** — 骨化〔症〕
  - ectopic ossification — 異所性骨化
  - ossification of posterior longitudinal ligament (OPLL) — 後縦（こうじゅう）靭帯骨化症
- polymyalgia rheumatica (PMR) — リウマチ性多〔発性〕筋痛〔症〕

1	☐ polymyositis	多発〔性〕筋炎
2	☐ polymyositis/dermatomyositis	多発〔性〕筋炎 / 皮膚筋炎
3	(PM/DM)	
4	☐ **rupture**	**破裂，断裂**
5	☐ Achilles tendon rupture	アキレス腱断裂
6	☐ **stiff neck and shoulder**	**肩こり**
7	☐ tendonitis	腱炎
8	☐ **tenosynovitis; tendovaginitis**	**腱鞘炎**
9	☐ stenosing tenosynovitis	狭窄性腱鞘炎

2-4. Movements and Gaits　運動・歩行

12	☐ **contraction**	**収縮**
13	☐ isometric contraction	等尺性収縮
14	☐ isotonic contraction	等張性収縮
15	☐ dyskinesia	ジスキネジア，運動異常症，運動障害
17	☐ **immobilization**	**固定，不動化**
18	☐ Jacksonian seizure	ジャクソン型発作
19	☐ **gait**	**歩行**
20	☐ abnormal gait	異常歩行
21	☐ alternating three-point gait	交互式三点歩行
22	☐ always two-point support gait	常時二点支持歩行，三点〔動作〕歩行
23	☐ calcaneal gait	踵足歩行
24	☐ circumduction gait	分回し歩行
25	☐ crutch gait	松葉杖歩行
26	☐ equinovarus gait	内反尖足歩行
27	☐ four-point gait	四点歩行
28	☐ gait disturbance	歩行障害
29	☐ gait on heels	踵歩き
30	☐ gluteus maximus gait	大殿筋歩行，股関節伸展筋歩行

1	☐ gluteus medius gait	中殿筋歩行
2	☐ independent gait	独歩
3	☐ intermittent claudication	間欠性跛行（はこう）
4	☐ scissors gait	はさみ歩行
5	☐ shuffle alternate gait	交互ひきずり歩行
6	☐ shuffle simultaneous gait	同時ひきずり歩行
7	☐ steppage gait	鶏歩
8	☐ swing-through gait	大振り歩行
9	☐ swing-to gait	小振り歩行
10	☐ three-point gait	三点歩行
11	☐ Trendelenburg gait	トレンデレンブルグ歩行
12	☐ two and one point gait	二点一点歩行，二点一点交互
13		支持（二動作）歩行
14	☐ vaulting gait	伸び上がり歩行
15	☐ waddling gait	アヒル歩行
16	☐ **mobility**	**可動性**
17	☐ mobility impairment	運動障害
18	☐ **motion**	**運動**《動き，動作》
19	☐ range of motion (ROM)	可動域
20	☐ **movement**	**運動**《動かすこと》
21	☐ associated movement	連合運動
22	☐ athetoid movement	アテトーゼ様運動
23	☐ dystonic movement	ジストニー運動
24	☐ involuntary movement	不随運動

Part 2 **Medical Terms** 医学・医療の基本英単語

3 Diseases and Disorders of the Circulatory System 循環器系の疾患・障害

3-1. Heart 心臓

- **angina pectoris (AP);** precordial anxiety; stenocardia — **狭心症；前胸[部]苦悶[症]**
- ☐ aortic atresia — 大動脈弁閉鎖[症]
- ☐ aortic insufficiency; aortic regurgitation — 大動脈弁閉鎖不全[症]；大動脈弁逆流[症]
- **arrhythmia;** abnormal heart rhythm — **不整脈**
- ☐ bradycardia — 徐脈
- ☐ cardiac amyloidosis — 心アミロイドーシス
- **cardiac arrest** — **心停止**
- ☐ cardiac tumor — 心臓腫瘍
- **cardiomyopathy (CM)** — **心筋症**
  - ☐ arrhythmogenic right ventricular cardiomyopathy (ARVCM) — 不整脈原性右室心筋症
  - ☐ congestive cardiomyopathy (CCM; COCM) — うっ血型心筋症
  - ☐ dilated cardiomyopathy (DCM) — 拡張型心筋症
  - ☐ hypertrophic cardiomyopathy (HCM) — 肥大型心筋症
  - ☐ restrictive cardiomyopathy (RCM) — 拘束型心筋症
- ☐ cor pulmonale — 肺性心
- ☐ coronary artery disease (CAD) — 冠[状]動脈[性心]疾患
- ☐ coronary heart disease (CHD) — 冠[状]動脈[性]心疾患
- ☐ endocarditis — 心内膜炎
  - ☐ infective endocarditis — 感染性心内膜炎
- **heart failure;** cardic insufficiency — **心不全**
  - ☐ congestive heart failure (CHF) — うっ血性心不全
- ☐ heart septal defect — 心臓中隔欠損[症]

1	☐ atrial septal defect (ASD)	心房中隔欠損〔症〕
2	☐ ventricular septal defect (VSD)	心室中隔欠損〔症〕
3	☐ **ischemic heart disease (IHD)**	**虚血性心疾患**
4	☐ mitral stenosis	僧帽弁狭窄症
5	☐ **myocardial infarction (MI);**	**心筋梗塞〔症〕；心臓発作**
6	**heart attack**	
7	☐ myocarditis	心筋炎
8	☐ pericarditis	心外膜炎
9	☐ postpericardiotomy syndrome	心〔膜〕切開後症候群
10	☐ sudden cardiac death (SCD)	心臓突然死
11	☐ **tachycardia**	**頻脈**
12	☐ valvular heart disease	心臓弁膜症

3-2. Blood Vessels　　　　血管系

15	☐ **aneurysm**	**動脈瘤**
16	☐ aortic aneurysm	大動脈瘤
17	☐ **angitis; angiitis**	**血管炎**
18	☐ allergic granulomatous angitis (AGA);	アレルギー性肉芽腫血管炎；
19	Churg-Strauss syndrome (CSS)	チャーグ-ストラウス症候群
20	☐ hypersensitivity angitis	過敏性血管炎
21	☐ **arteriosclerosis**	**動脈硬化〔症〕**
22	☐ arteriosclerosis obliterans (ASO)	閉塞性動脈硬化〔症〕
23	☐ **arteritis**	**動脈炎**
24	☐ giant cell arteritis (GCA)	巨細胞動脈炎
25	☐ Takayasu arteritis; aortitis syndrome;	高安動脈炎；大動脈炎症候群；
26	pulseless disease	脈なし病
27	☐ temporal arteritis (TA)	側頭動脈炎
28	☐ ataxia telangiectasia	毛細〔血〕管拡張性運動失調〔症〕
29	☐ **atherosclerosis**	**アテローム〔性動脈〕硬化〔症〕，粥状硬化〔症〕**

1	☐ atherothrombotic infarction	アテローム血栓性梗塞〔症〕
2	☐ bruit; vascular murmur	血管雑音《断続性聴診音》
3	☐ Budd-Chiari syndrome	バッド-キアリ症候群
4	☐ Buerger disease; thromboangiitis obliterans	ビュルガー(バージャー)病；閉塞性血栓血管炎
6	☐ hemochromatosis	ヘモクロマトーシス
7	☐ **hypertension**; **high blood pressure**	高血圧〔症〕
9	☐ pulmonary hypertension (PH)	肺高血圧〔症〕
10	☐ **hypotension**; **low blood pressure**	低血圧〔症〕
11	☐ orthostatic hypotension	起立性低血圧〔症〕
12	☐ Kawasaki disease; mucocutaneous lymph node syndrome (MCLS)	川崎病；皮膚粘膜リンパ節症候群
14	☐ phlebitis	静脈炎
15	☐ polyangiitis	多発〔性〕血管炎
16	☐ micoroscopic polyangiitis (MPR)	顕微鏡的多発血管炎
17	☐ polyarteritis	多発〔性〕動脈炎
18	☐ polyarteritis nodosa (PN)	結節性多発〔性〕動脈炎
19	☐ Raynaud syndrome	レーノー(レイノー)症候群
20	☐ thrombophlebitits	血栓性静脈炎
21	☐ varix	静脈瘤
22	☐ esophageal varix	食道静脈瘤
23	☐ lower extremity varix	下肢静脈瘤
24	☐ vasculitis syndrome	血管炎症候群

4 Diseases and Disorders of the Nervous System 脳神経系の疾患・障害

4-1. Brain 脳

- [ ] acalculia — 失算症
- [ ] agnosia — 失認〔症〕，認知不能〔症〕
- [ ] finger agnosia — 手指失認〔症〕
- [ ] object agnosia — 物体失認〔症〕
- [ ] unilateral spatial neglect (agnosia) — 半側空間無視（失認）
- [ ] visual agnosia — 視覚失認〔症〕
- [ ] visuospatial agnosia — 視空間失認〔症〕
- [ ] agrammatism — 失文法〔症〕
- [ ] agraphia — 失書〔症〕
- [ ] alexia — 失読〔症〕
- [ ] pure alexia — 純粋失読〔症〕
- [ ] **Alzheimer disease** — **アルツハイマー病**
- [ ] anarthria — 失構語〔症〕，構音不能〔症〕
- [ ] anosognosia — 病態失認〔症〕
- [ ] apathy — 感情鈍麻，無関心
- [ ] **aphasia** — **失語〔症〕**
- [ ] amnestic aphasia — 健忘失語〔症〕
- [ ] Broca aphasia — ブローカ失語〔症〕
- [ ] Wernicke aphasia — ウェルニッケ失語〔症〕
- [ ] aphonia — 失声〔症〕
- [ ] **apraxia** — **失行〔症〕**
- [ ] buccofacial apraxia — 口腔顔面失行〔症〕
- [ ] constructional apraxia — 構成失行〔症〕
- [ ] dressing apraxia — 着衣失行〔症〕
- [ ] idiomotor apraxia — 観念運動性失行〔症〕
- [ ] limb kinetic apraxia — 肢節運動失行〔症〕

	☐ **ataxia**	〔運動〕失調〔症〕
	☐ **brain concussion**; cerebral concussion	脳震盪（のうしんとう）
	☐ brain contusion; cerebral contusion	脳挫傷
	☐ brain tumor; cerebral tumor	脳腫瘍
	☐ cerebral embolism	脳塞栓〔症〕
	☐ **cerebral hemorrhage**	**脳内出血**
	☐ **cerebral (brain) infarction**	**脳梗塞〔症〕**
	☐ cerebral thrombosis	脳血栓〔症〕
	☐ cerebrovascular disorder (CVD)	脳血管障害
	☐ **cervical cord injury**	**頚髄損傷**
	☐ **disorientation**	**見当識障害**
	☐ dysarthria; articulation disorder	構音障害
	☐ **encephalitis**	**脳炎**
	☐ herpes simplex encephalitis (HSE)	単純ヘルペス脳炎
	☐ encephalopathy	脳症
	☐ toxic encephalopathy	中毒性脳症
	☐ higher brain dysfunction	高次脳機能障害
	☐ ischemic cerebrovascular disease	虚血性脳血管障害
	☐ late cerebellar cortical atrophy (LCCA)	晩発性小脳皮質萎縮症
	☐ meningioma	髄膜腫
	☐ **meningitis**	**髄膜炎**
	☐ pneumonococcal meningitis	肺炎球菌性髄膜炎
	☐ **migraine**	**片(偏)頭痛**
	☐ **Parkinson disease**	**パーキンソン病**
	☐ Pick disease	ピック病《進行性限局性脳萎縮》
	☐ Rye syndrome	ライ症候群
	☐ simultanagnosia	同時失認

1	☐ speech disorder (impediment)	言語障害，発話障害
2	☐ **stroke**	**脳卒中**
3	☐ cerebrovascular accident (stroke) (CVA)	脳血管障害，脳卒中
4	☐ **subarachnoidal hemorrhage (SAH)**	**くも膜下出血**
5	☐ **subdural hematoma**	**硬膜下血腫**
6	☐ subdural hemorrhage	硬膜下出血
7	☐ transient ischemic attack (TIA)	一過性脳虚血発作
8	☐ traumatic brain injury (TBI)	脳外傷，外傷性脳損傷
9	☐ **tremor**	**振戦，震顫（しんせん）**
10	☐ cerebellar tremor	小脳性振戦

4-2. Nervous System　　　　　　神経系

13	☐ athetosis	アテトーゼ
14	☐ autonomous (hypernomic) hyperreflexia	自律神経過〔緊張〕反射
16	☐ brachial plexopathy	腕神経叢障害
17	☐ **carpal tunnel syndrome**	**手根管症候群**
18	☐ cataplexy	カタプレキシー，脱力発作
19	☐ causalgia	カウザルギー，灼熱痛
20	☐ central coordination disorder; Zentrale Koordinationsstörung (ZKS)	中枢性協調障害
22	☐ **chronic fatigue syndrome (CFS)**	**慢性疲労症候群**
23	☐ **chorea**	**舞踏病**
24	☐ Huntington disease (chorea)	ハンチントン病（舞踏病）
25	☐ Sydenham chorea; rheumatic chorea	シデナム舞踏病；リウマチ性舞踏病
26	☐ Creutzfeldt-Jakob disease (CJD)	クロイツフェルト−ヤコブ病
27	☐ diffuse axonal injury (DAI)	びまん性軸索損傷
28	☐ diplegia	両麻痺
29	☐ encephalomyelitis	脳脊髄炎
30	☐ focal motor seizure	焦点〔運動〕発作

□	Froment sign	フロマン徴候
□	glioma	神経膠腫
□	Guillain-Barré syndrome (GBS)	ギラン(ギヤン)-バレー症候群
□	hemifacial spasm	片側顔面れん(攣)縮
□	**hemiplegia**	**片(へん)麻痺**
□	hemiplegia cruciata	交差片麻痺
□	Ménierè disease	メニエール病
□	monoplegia	単麻痺
□	moyamoya disease; Nishimoto-Takeuchi-Kudo disease	もやもや病；西本－竹内－工藤病
□	multiple system atrophy (MSA)	多系統萎縮症
□	myelitis	脊髄炎
□	myelopathy	脊髄障害，脊髄症
□	HTLV-1 associated myelopathy (HAM)	HTLV-1関連脊髄症
□	myoclonus	ミオクローヌス
□	narcolepsy	ナルコレプシー，睡眠発作
□	**neuralgia**	**神経痛**
□	trigeminal neuralgia	三叉神経痛
□	neurapraxia	ニューラプラキシア
□	neurofibroma	神経線維腫
□	**neuropathy**	**ニューロパチー**
□	entrapment neuropathy	エントラップメント(絞扼性)ニューロパチー
□	idiopathic peripheral autonomic neuropathy	特発性末梢性自律神経ニューロパチー
□	peripheral neuropathy	末梢神経障害
□	olive-ponto-cerebellar atrophy (OPCA)	オリーブ橋小脳萎縮症
□	**palsy**	**麻痺**
□	athetotic type palsy	アテトーシス型麻痺
□	bilateral spastic cerebral palsy	両側性痙性脳性麻痺

1	☐ brachial plexus palsy	腕神経叢麻痺
2	☐ bulbar palsy	球麻痺
3	☐ cerebral [infantile] palsy (CP)	脳性〔小児〕麻痺
4	☐ musculocutaneous nerve palsy	筋皮神経麻痺
5	☐ peroneal (fibular) nerve palsy	腓骨神経麻痺
6	☐ radial nerve palsy	橈骨(とうこつ)神経麻痺
7	☐ ulnar nerve palsy	尺骨神経麻痺
8	☐ **paralysis**	**〔完全〕麻痺**
9	☐ facial paralysis	顔面神経麻痺
10	☐ flaccid paralysis	弛緩性麻痺
11	☐ motor paralysis	運動麻痺
12	☐ paralysis of the brachial plexus	腕神経叢麻痺
13	☐ **paraparesis**	**不全対麻痺**
14	☐ tropical spastic paraparesis (TSP)	熱帯性痙性不全対麻痺
15	☐ paraplegia	対麻痺
16	☐ paresis	不全麻痺
17	☐ paresthesia	感覚異常
18	☐ periodic limb movement disorder (PLMD)	周期性四肢運動障害
20	☐ **poliomyelitis; polio**	**灰白髄炎；ポリオ**
21	☐ acute anterior poliomyelitis	急性灰白髄炎
22	☐ postviral fatigue syndrome	ウイルス感染後疲弊症候群
23	☐ pyramidal tract disorder	錐体路障害
24	☐ quadriplegia	四肢麻痺
25	☐ reversible ischemic neurological deficits (RIND)	可逆性虚血性神経脱落症状
27	☐ sciatica; sciatic neuralgia	坐骨神経痛
28	☐ **sclerosis**	**硬化症**
29	☐ amyotrophic lateral sclerosis (ALS); Lou Gehrig disease	筋萎縮性側索硬化症：ルー・ゲーリッグ病

☐	multiple sclerosis (MS)	多発〔性〕硬化〔症〕
☐	simian hand; ape hand	猿手（さるて）
☐	spinal cord disease (SCD)	脊髄疾患
☐	**spinal cord injury (SCI)**	**脊髄損傷**
☐	high spinal cord injury	高位脊髄損傷
☐	lumbar spinal cord injury	腰髄損傷
☐	thoracic spinal cord injury	胸髄損傷
☐	syringomyelia	脊髄空洞症
☐	tarsal tunnel syndrome (TTS)	足根管症候群
☐	triplegia	三肢麻痺
☐	vasovagal syndrome	血管迷走神経症候群
☐	vegetative dystonia	自律神経失調症

5 Diseases and Disorders of the Sense Organs and Throat 感覚器官の疾患・障害

5-1. Eye 眼

- amblyopia; lazy eye 弱視
- anisometropia 不同視
- asthenopia; eyestrain 眼精疲労；疲れ目
- astigmatism 乱視
- blepharoptosis 眼瞼下垂
- blindness 盲, 失明
- color blindness; dyschromatopsia 色弱；色覚異常
- cortical blindness 皮質盲
- day blindness; hemeralopia 昼盲〔症〕
- night blindness; nocturnal amblyopia; nyctalopia 夜盲〔症〕
- **cataract** 白内障
- **choroiditis** 脈絡膜炎
- acute diffuse choroiditis; Harada disease; Vogt-Koyanagi-Harada disease 急性びまん性脈絡膜炎；原田病；フォークト－小柳－原田病
- **conjunctivitis** 結膜炎
- atopic conjunctivitis アトピー性結膜炎
- corneal xerosis 角膜乾燥症
- cross-eyed 斜視の
- dacryocystitis 涙嚢炎
- diplopia; double vision 複視
- dry eye syndrome; keratoconjunctivitis sicca; keratitis sicca ドライアイ症候群；乾性角結膜炎
- dyschromatopsia; color vision deficiency; color vision defect 色覚異常
- exophthalmos; exophthalmus 眼球突出

Part 2 **Medical Terms** 医学・医療の基本英単語

☐ eye mucus	目脂(めやに)
☐ flying flies; myodesopsia	飛蚊症(ひぶんしょう)
☐ **glaucoma**	**緑内障**
☐ hyperopia; hypermetropia; far-sightedness	遠視
☐ keratitis	角膜炎
☐ **keratoconjunctivitis**	**角結膜炎**
☐ epidemic keratoconjunctivitis (EKC); pink eye	流行性角結膜炎:はやり目
☐ keratopathy	角膜症
☐ bullous keratopathy	水疱性角膜症
☐ lacrimal passage obstruction; dacryostenosis	涙道閉塞症(狭窄)
☐ lagophthalmos	兎眼
☐ **macular degeneration**	**黄斑変性症**
☐ age-related macular degeneration (AMD)	加齢黄斑変性症
☐ maculopathy	黄斑症
☐ misty vision	霧視(むし)
☐ myopia; near-sightedness	近視
☐ nystagmus blockage syndrome	眼振遮断症候群《斜視の一種》
☐ optic ataxia	視覚失調
☐ photophobia; photoalgia	光恐怖〔症〕;光痛〔症〕
☐ photosensitivity	羞明(しゅうめい), 光線過敏症
☐ presbyopia; old-sightedness	老視, 老眼
☐ **retinopathy**	**網膜症**
☐ diabetic retinopathy (DR)	糖尿病〔性〕網膜症
☐ strabismus; heterotropia; squint	斜視
☐ sty; hordeolum	ものもらい:麦粒腫
☐ uveitis	ブドウ膜炎
☐ visual distortion	歪曲視

- ☐ visual filed defect　　　　　視野欠損
- ☐ visual impairment　　　　　視力障害，視力低下

5-2. Ear　　　　　耳

- ☐ acoustic trauma　　　　　音響外傷
- ☐ acoustic tumor　　　　　聴神経腫瘍
- ☐ anacusis　　　　　聴覚消失症
- ☐ auditory agnosia　　　　　聴覚失認
- ☐ auditory fatigue　　　　　聴覚疲労
- ☐ auditory hallucination　　　　　幻聴
- ☐ cerumen; earwax　　　　　耳垢(じこう)
- ☐ cerumen impaction; impacted cerumen　　　　　耳垢栓塞
- ☐ **deafness**　　　　　**聴覚障害，難聴，聴覚消失，ろう(聾)**
  - ☐ perceptive deafness; sensorineural deafness　　　　　感音性難聴
  - ☐ pure word deafness　　　　　純粋語ろう
- ☐ ear discharge　　　　　耳漏
- ☐ ear noise; tinnitus; susurrus aurium　　　　　耳鳴り
- ☐ hearing loss; hearing impairment; difficulty in hearing　　　　　聴覚消失；聴覚障害，難聴
  - ☐ conductive hearing loss　　　　　伝音性難聴
  - ☐ high frequency hearing loss　　　　　高音域障害
  - ☐ idiopathic sudden sensorineural hearing impairment; sudden deafness　　　　　突発性難聴
  - ☐ noise-induced hearing loss　　　　　騒音性難聴
- ☐ mastoiditis　　　　　乳〔様〕突〔起〕炎
- ☐ myringitis　　　　　鼓膜炎
- ☐ otalgia; ear pain; otodynia　　　　　耳痛

1	☐ **otitis externa**; external otitis	外耳炎
2	☐ **otitis interna**; internal otitis	内耳炎
3	☐ **otitis media**; medial otitis	中耳炎
4	☐ cholesteatomatous otitis media	真珠腫性中耳炎
5	☐ secretory otitis media; serous otitis media (SOM)	滲出性中耳炎
7	☐ otosclerosis	耳硬化症
8	☐ **parotiditis**	**耳下腺炎**
9	☐ residual hearing	残聴
10	☐ traumatic eardrum perforation	外傷性鼓膜穿孔，鼓膜破裂
11	☐ tubal obstruction; plugged ear	耳管閉塞症；耳詰まり
12	☐ tubal stenosis	耳管狭窄症

5-3. Nose and Throat　　　　　鼻・咽喉

15	☐ anosmia	無嗅覚，嗅覚消失
16	☐ dysosmia; olfactory disturbance	嗅覚障害
17	☐ dysphonia	発声障害
18	☐ epipharyngitis	上咽頭炎
19	☐ acute epipharyngitis	急性上咽頭炎
20	☐ hyposmia	嗅覚鈍麻
21	☐ laryngeal cancer	喉頭がん
22	☐ laryngeal polyp	喉頭ポリープ
23	☐ **laryngitis**	**喉頭炎**
24	☐ nasal furuncle	鼻癤（びせつ）
25	☐ nasal hemorrhage; epistaxis; nosebleed	鼻出血；鼻血
27	☐ nasal polyp; rhinopolypus	鼻ポリープ；鼻茸（はなたけ）
28	☐ nasal reflex-neurosis	鼻性反射神経症
29	☐ nasopharyngitis	鼻咽頭炎
30	☐ acute nasopharyngitis	急性鼻咽頭炎，かぜ

1	☐ olfactory hyperesthesia	嗅覚過敏
2	☐ **pharyngitis**	**咽頭炎**
3	☐ **rhinitis**	**鼻炎**
4	☐ allergic rhinitis; pollenosis	アレルギー性鼻炎；花粉症
5	☐ vasomotor rhinitis	血管運動性鼻炎
6	☐ septal deviation	鼻中隔弯曲症
7	☐ **sinusitis**	**副鼻腔炎，蓄膿症**
8	☐ tonsillitis	〔口蓋〕扁桃炎
9	☐ vocal cord paralysis; vocal cord palsy	声帯麻痺
11	☐ vocal nodule	声帯結節

5-4. Skin　　皮膚

14	☐ **acne**	**痤瘡(ざそう)，にきび**
15	☐ acne vulgaris	尋常性痤瘡
16	☐ alopecia; calvities; baldness	脱毛〔症〕；禿頭〔症〕；はげ《毛髪がないこと》
18	☐ alopecia areate	円形脱毛症
19	☐ atrophoderma; atrophia cutis; dermatrophia	皮膚萎縮；末端肥大症《皮膚の萎縮》
21	☐ Behçet disease	ベーチェット病
22	☐ bulla; blister	水疱《皮膚下の水膨れ》
23	☐ bullous pemphigoid	水疱性類天疱瘡
24	☐ burn; burn injury	やけど，熱傷
25	☐ carbuncle	癰(よう)，カルブンケル
26	☐ cellulitis	蜂巣炎，フレグモーネ，小胞炎
27	☐ chloasma	肝斑，しみ
28	☐ chronic mucocutaneous candidiasis (CMC)	慢性粘膜皮膚カンジダ症
30	☐ crust	痂皮(かひ)

1	☐ decubital ulcer; bedsore	じょく(褥)瘡〔性潰瘍〕；床ずれ
2	☐ depigmentation	色素脱失
3	☐ **dermatitis**	**皮膚炎**
4	☐ atopic dermatitis; atopic eczema	アトピー性皮膚炎；アトピー性湿疹
6	☐ contact dermatitis	接触皮膚炎
7	☐ solar dermatitis	日光皮膚炎
8	☐ dermatonecrosis	皮膚壊死
9	☐ dermatosis	皮膚症
10	☐ chronic bullous dermatosis of children; linear IgA bullous disease in children	小児慢性水疱症；〔小児期〕線状IgA水疱性皮膚症
13	☐ **eczema**	**湿疹**
14	☐ elastosis	弾性線維症
15	☐ epidermolysis bullosa acquisita (EBA)	後天性表皮水疱症
16	☐ **eruption; rash**	**発疹，皮疹**
17	☐ drug eruption; drug rash; medical eruption	薬疹
19	☐ butterfly rash	蝶形紅斑
20	☐ **erythema; rubor**	**紅斑，発赤(ほっせき)**
21	☐ erythema infectiosum; fifth disease	伝染性紅斑；第五病，りんご病
22	☐ erythema multiforme bullosum; Stevens-Johnson syndrome	多形水疱性紅斑；スティーブンス-ジョンソン症候群
24	☐ toxic erythema; erythema toxicum	中毒性紅斑
25	☐ erythralgia	皮膚紅痛症
26	☐ furuncle; boil	癤(せつ)，フルンケル；おでき
27	☐ furunculosis	癤(せつ)多発症，フルンケル多発症，癤腫症
29	☐ heliophobia	日光恐怖症
30	☐ hirsuitism; hypertrichosis	〔男性型〕多毛

1	☐ ichthyosis vulgaris	尋常性魚鱗癬(ぎょりんせん)
2	☐ Kaposi sarcoma; multiple idiopathic hemorrhagic sarcoma	カポジ肉腫；特発性多発性出血性肉腫
4	☐ leukoderma	白斑
5	☐ leukoderma acquisitum centrifugum; Sutton nevus	遠心性後天性白斑；サットン母斑
7	☐ **melanoma**	**黒色腫，メラノーマ**
8	☐ nevus; birthmark	母斑，あざ
9	☐ papule; pimple	丘疹
10	☐ pemphigus	天疱瘡
11	☐ pigmentation; chromatosis	色素沈着
12	☐ **pruritus**	**瘙痒症**
13	☐ **psoriasis**	**乾癬**
14	☐ psoriasis arthropica	関節性乾癬
15	☐ **purpura**	**紫斑〔病〕**
16	☐ allergic purpura; Henoch-Schönlein purpura	アレルギー性紫斑症；ヘーノホーシェーンライン紫斑症
18	☐ rose spot	バラ疹
19	☐ **scabies**	**疥癬**
20	☐ **scleroderma; erythrodema**	**強皮症；紅皮症**
21	☐ diffuse scleroderma; progressive systemic sclerosis (PSS); systemic screroderma (SS)	汎発性全身硬化症；進行性全身性強皮(硬化)症；全身性強皮(硬化)症
24	☐ locarized scleroderma; circumscribed scleroderma	限局性強皮症
26	☐ staphylococcal scalded skin syndrome (SSSS)	ブドウ球菌性熱傷様皮膚症候群
28	☐ stiff skin	皮膚硬化
29	☐ tinea pedis; athlete's foot	汗疱状白癬；水虫
30	☐ **urticaria; hives; nettle rush**	**蕁麻疹(じんましん)**

1	☐ verruca; wart	疣贅（ゆうぜい）；いぼ
2	☐ vitiligo	尋常性白斑，白なまず
3	☐ xeroderma	乾皮症
4	☐ xeroderma pigmentosum (XP)	色素性乾皮症

COLUMN 痛みはさまざま

痛みは病気の徴候の1つであり，その程度を知る重要な指標となる。そして，患者はあらゆる個所の痛みを，さまざまな表現で訴える。

それらを英語で覚えるのもかなり pain in the neck（悩みの種）であるが，ひとまず知っておきたいもの。

1. 痛みの違い

ache：痛みの局在が明確でない。長く続く鈍痛。心身の痛み。
pain：身体局部的で鋭い痛み。疼痛。陣痛。
sore：圧痛。触痛。けがや炎症による痛み。
stiff：凝った筋肉痛。関節を動かすときの痛み。
tenderness：圧痛，触痛。
anguish, distress, sorrow, worry：心の痛み

2. 程度を表す表現

acute / chronic：急性 / 慢性
severe / mild：ひどい，重症 / 軽度
persistent / intermittent：持続的 / 間欠的

3. 性質を表す表現

burning：ひりひりする　　gripping：きりきりする
penetrating：差し込むような　piercing：刺すような
prickling：ちくちくする　　shooting：うずくような
splitting：割れるような　　throbbing：ずきずきする

今，"I have a pain in my head" と声が聞えたような。"No pain, no gain."（苦労しないと得るものもない）のであるから，"I don't care at all about any pain."（痛みもなんのその）と言ってほしい。

6 Diseases and Disorders of the Respiratory System 呼吸器系の疾患・障害

- □ **adult respiratory distress syndrome (ARDS)** 成人呼吸窮迫（促迫）症候群
- □ **apnea** 無呼吸
- □ **asthma** 喘息
  - □ allergic asthma アレルギー性喘息
  - □ bronchial asthma 気管支喘息
- □ bronchial ectasia; bronchiectasis (BE) 気管支拡張症
- □ **bronchitis** 気管支炎
- □ bronchogenic carcinoma 気管支原性〔肺〕がん
- □ **chronic obstructive pulmonary disease (COPD)** 慢性閉塞性肺疾患
- □ croup クループ
- □ **dyspnea** 呼吸困難
- □ **emphysema** 気腫
  - □ interstitial emphysema 間質性気腫
  - □ pulmonary emphysema 肺気腫
- □ hyperventilation syndrome 過換気症候群, 過呼吸症候群
- □ lung cancer 肺がん
- □ lymphangiomyomatosis (LAM) リンパ脈管筋腫症
  - □ pulmonary lymphangiomyomatosis 肺リンパ脈管筋腫症
- □ mediastinal tumor 縦隔腫瘍
- □ obstructive ventilator disturbance 閉塞性換気障害
- □ orthopnea 起座呼吸
- □ pleural mesothelioma 胸膜中皮腫
- □ pleurisy; pleuritis 胸膜炎
  - □ purulent (suppurative) pleurisy 化膿性胸膜炎

1	☐ **pneumonia**	**肺炎**
2	☐ bronchial pneumonia	気管支肺炎
3	☐ chlamydial pneumonia	クラミジア肺炎
4	☐ eosinophilic pneumonia; PIE (pulmonary	好酸球性肺炎；PIE（肺好酸球
5	infiltration with eosinophilia) syndrome	浸潤）症候群
6	☐ interstitial pneumonia	間質性肺炎
7	☐ pneumonitis	肺〔臓〕炎
8	☐ hypersensitivity pneumonitis	過敏性肺〔臓〕炎
9	☐ pneumonoconiosis	塵肺症
10	☐ **pneumothorax**	**気胸**
11	☐ spontaneous pneumothorax	自然気胸
12	☐ polypnea	多呼吸
13	☐ postprocedual respiratory disorder	処置後呼吸器障害
14	☐ pulmonary edema	肺水腫
15	☐ pulmonary embolism	肺塞栓〔症〕
16	☐ pulmonary thromboembolism	肺血栓塞栓症
17	☐ **respiratory failure**	**呼吸不全**
18	☐ respiratory paralysis	呼吸麻痺
19	☐ **severe acute respiratory**	**重症急性呼吸器症候群**
20	**syndrome (SARS)**	
21	☐ **sleep apnea syndrome (SAS)**	**睡眠時無呼吸症候群**
22	☐ tachypnea	頻呼吸
23	☐ **tuberculosis (TB); pulmonary**	**〔肺〕結核**
24	**tuberculosis**	
25	☐ unilateral lobar emphysema	片側性透過性亢進肺

7 Diseases and Disorders of the Digestive System
消化器系の疾患・障害

1. ☐ abdominal pain; bellyache — 腹痛
2. ☐ acalasia — アカラシア
3. ☐ anal fissure — 裂肛
4. ☐ anal fistula — 痔瘻(ろう)
5. ☐ anal prolapse — 脱肛
6. ☐ **appendicitis** — **虫垂炎**
7. ☐ celiac disease; gluten enteropathy — シェリアキー，セリアック
8. 病；グルテン性腸症
9. ☐ cholecystitis — 胆嚢炎
10. ☐ choledocholithiasis — 総胆管結石症
11. ☐ cholangitis — 胆管炎
12. ☐ cholelithiasis; cholelith — 胆石症；胆石
13. ☐ **cirrhosis** — **肝硬変**
14. ☐ primary biliary cirrhosis — 原発性胆汁性肝硬変
15. ☐ **colitis** — **大腸炎**
16. ☐ ulcerative colitis (UC) — 潰瘍性大腸炎
17. ☐ colon cancer — 大腸がん，結腸がん
18. ☐ **constipation** — **便秘**
19. ☐ Crohn disease; regional enteritis — クローン病；限局性腸炎
20. ☐ **diarrhea; loose stool** — **下痢**
21. ☐ duodenal cancer — 十二指腸がん
22. ☐ **duodenal ulcer** — **十二指腸潰瘍**
23. ☐ duodenitis — 十二指腸炎
24. ☐ dysphagia — 嚥下(えんげ)障害，嚥下困難
25. ☐ enteritis — 腸炎
26. ☐ enterocele — 脱腸
27. ☐ esophageal carcinoma — 食道がん

1	☐ esophageal reflux	食道逆流
2	☐ **esophagitis**	**食道炎**
3	☐ fatty liver	脂肪肝
4	☐ flank pain	側腹痛
5	☐ gallbladder cancer	胆嚢がん
6	☐ gastric cancer; stomach cancer	胃がん
7	☐ gastric hyperacidity	胃酸過多
8	☐ gastric subacidity	胃酸減少
9	☐ **gastritis**	**胃炎**
10	☐ reflux gastritis	逆流性胃炎
11	☐ gastric diverticulum	胃憩室
12	☐ **gastric ulcer**	**胃潰瘍**
13	☐ gastroenteritis	胃腸炎
14	☐ gastroenteropathy	胃腸症
15	☐ **gastroesophageal reflux disease (GERD)**	**胃食道逆流性疾患**
17	☐ gastroptosis	胃下垂
18	☐ hemorrhoid; pile	痔核
19	☐ hepatic failure	肝不全
20	☐ **hepatitis**	**肝炎**
21	☐ hepatocellular carcinoma (HCC); hepatocarcinoma; liver cell carcinoma	肝細胞がん
23	☐ hepatomegaly	肝腫大
24	☐ hepatopathy	肝障害
25	☐ alcoholic hepatopathy; alcoholic liver disease	アルコール性肝障害
27	☐ hereditary nonpolyposis colorectal cancer (HNPCC); Lynch syndrome; cancer family syndrome	遺伝性非ポリポーシス大腸がん；リンチ症候群；がん家族症候群
30	☐ hiatal hernia	裂孔ヘルニア

2 医学・医療の基本英単語

1	☐ hypogastalgia; lower abdominal pain	下腹部痛
2	☐ ileus; intestinal obstruction	イレウス；腸閉塞〔症〕
3	☐ adynamic ileus; paralytic ileus	麻痺性イレウス（腸麻痺）
4	☐ **inflammatory bowel disease (IBD)**	**炎症性腸疾患**
5	☐ indigestion; dyspepsia	消化不良
6	☐ inguinal hernia	鼡径ヘルニア
7	☐ intrahepatic bile duct cancer;	肝内胆管がん；胆管細胞がん
8	cholangiocellular carcinoma	
9	☐ liver cancer	肝〔臓〕がん
10	☐ megacolon	巨大結腸症
11	☐ melena; tarry stool	メレナ；タール様便（黒色便）
12	☐ pancreatic cancer	膵〔臓〕がん
13	☐ **pancreatitis**	**膵〔臓〕炎**
14	☐ peptic ulcer	消化性潰瘍
15	☐ peritonitis	腹膜炎
16	☐ portal hypertension	門脈圧亢進症
17	☐ postgastroectomy syndrome	胃切除後症候群
18	☐ rectal cancer	直腸がん
19	☐ rectosigmoid cancer	直腸S状結腸がん

7-1. Dentistry / Oral Surgery　　歯科・口腔外科

22	☐ alveolitis; odontobothritis	歯槽炎
23	☐ canker sore; stomatitis	口内炎
24	☐ **carious tooth**; **dental caries**;	**う（齲）歯**：<u>虫歯</u>
25	**dental decay**	
26	☐ gingival bleeding	歯肉出血
27	☐ **gingivitis**	**歯肉炎**
28	☐ glossitis	舌炎
29	☐ lingual cancer; tongue cancer	舌がん
30	☐ malocculusion	不正咬合

Part 2 **Medical Terms** 医学・医療の基本英単語

- [ ] maxillary cancer 　　　　　　上顎がん
- [ ] oral aphtha 　　　　　　　　口腔アフタ
- [x] **periodontal disease** 　　　**歯周病**
- [ ] pharyngeal cancer 　　　　　咽頭がん
- [ ] pulpitis 　　　　　　　　　　歯髄炎
- [ ] salivary gland atrophy 　　　唾液腺萎縮
- [ ] salivary gland tumor; sialoma 　唾液腺腫瘍

COLUMN　病気になりそうな(？)病気の英語

diseaseとは，安らぎ(ease)が奪われた(dis-)状態をいう。さて，病気を表す語は他にもあり，各々微妙にニュアンスが違うのである。

- **disease**(疾患)：はっきりした病因と，徴候や症状があり，特定の病名がつく。
- **illness**：身体，精神が病気の状態。頭痛や風邪などは含めない。
- **sickness**：《米》身体の軽い病気の状態。《英》特定の病気のタイプ。
- **impairment**：体系，器官の構造・機能，心理的，生理的機能の障害，欠陥。
- **disorder**(障害)：身体的，精神的不調。遺伝，毒素，外傷，病気など外因性要因による。精神医学領域で使われることが多い。
- **disability**：能力の障害，身体の機能障害。
- **handicap**：社会的不利を伴う身体・精神上の障害。少し古い言い方で，侮蔑も含まれるので細菌ではdisabilityが好まれる。
- **syndrome**：症候群／シンドローム。いくつかの病的症状が組み合わさっており，原因や病理的所見が多岐にわたる。
- **dysfunction**：機能が異常，あるいは困難，不全である状態。

他にも，trouble, morbus, disturbanceなど。

"I feel sick at these words." とため息が出そうであるが，"Fancy may kill or cure." (気分は人を殺しもする)とも言うのだから。

8 Diseases and Disorders of the Genitourinary System　腎・尿路系の疾患・障害

1. ☐ bladder cancer　　膀胱がん
2. ☐ bladder papilloma　　膀胱乳頭がん
3. ☐ chronic kidney disease　　慢性腎臓病
4. ☐ cystic kidney disease　　嚢胞性腎疾患
5. ☐ **cystitis**　　**膀胱炎**
6. ☐ 　interstitial cystitis　　間質性膀胱炎
7. ☐ detrusor sphincter dyssynergia　　排尿筋－括約筋協調不全
8. 　　(DSD)
9. ☐ diabetes insipidus　　尿崩症
10. ☐ 　nephrogenic diabetes insipidus　　腎性尿崩症
11. ☐ dysuria　　排尿困難
12. ☐ ectopic ureter　　尿管異所開口
13. ☐ **glomerulonephritis**　　**糸球体腎炎**
14. ☐ 　membranoproliferative glomerulonephritis　　膜性増殖性糸球体腎炎
15. ☐ 　primary crescentic glomerulonephritis　　原発性半月体形成性糸球体腎炎
16. ☐ 　rapidly progressive glomerulonephritis　　急速進行性糸球体腎炎
17. 　　(RPGN)
18. ☐ Goodpasture syndrome　　グッドパスチャー症候群
19. ☐ **hematuria**　　**血尿**
20. ☐ hydronephrosis　　水腎症
21. ☐ lipiduria　　脂質尿症
22. ☐ micturition pain; miction pain　　排尿痛
23. ☐ **nephritis**　　**腎炎**
24. ☐ 　tubulointerstitial nephritis　　尿細管間質性腎炎
25. ☐ nephropathy　　腎症
26. ☐ 　IgA nephropathy; focal　　IgA腎症；巣状糸球体腎炎
27. 　　glomerulonephritis

□	nephrosclerosis	腎硬化症
□	diabetic nephrosclerosis	糖尿病性腎硬化症
□	**nephrosis**	**ネフローゼ**
□	nephrotic syndrome	ネフローゼ症候群
□	neurogenic bladder	神経因性膀胱炎，過敏膀胱
□	nocturia	夜間頻尿〔症〕
□	oliguria	乏尿〔症〕
□	pollakiuria; frequent urination	頻尿〔症〕
□	**polycystic kidney disease (PCKD, PKD)**	**多〔発性〕囊胞腎**
□	autosomal dominant polycystic kidney disease (ADPKD)	常染色体優性多囊胞腎
□	polyuria	多尿〔症〕
□	prostatic abscess	前立腺膿瘍
□	prostatic cancer	前立腺がん
□	**prostatic hyperplasia**	**前立腺肥大症**
□	benign prostatic hyperplasia (BPH)	良性前立腺肥大〔症〕
□	prostatic stone (calculus)	前立腺結石
□	prostatism	前立腺症
□	prostatitis	前立腺炎
□	prostatitis syndrome	前立腺炎症候群
□	prostatocystitis	前立腺膀胱炎
□	proteinuria	たんぱく（蛋白）尿
□	pyelonephritis	腎盂腎炎
□	pyonephrosis	膿腎症
□	pyuria	膿尿
□	renal amyloidosis	腎アミロイドーシス
□	renal carcinoma	腎〔臓〕がん
□	renal failure; end-stage renal disease (ESRD)	腎不全；末期腎疾患

	☐ chronic renal failure	慢性腎不全
	☐ renal infarction	腎梗塞
	☐ renal ischemia	腎虚血
	☐ renal calculus; kidney stone; nephrolith	腎〔結〕石
	☐ renal tubular acidosis	腎尿細管性アシドーシス
	☐ renal tubular dysfunction	腎尿細管不全
	☐ residual urine	残尿感
	☐ tubular necrosis	尿細管壊死
	☐ acute tubular necrosis	急性尿細管壊死
	☐ uremia	尿毒症
	☐ ureterolithiasis	尿管結石症
	☐ urethral stricture; urethral stenosis; urethrostenosis	尿道狭窄
	☐ urethral syndrome	尿道症候群
	☐ **urethritis**	**尿道炎**
	☐ gonococcal urethritis; gonorrheal urethritis	淋菌性尿道炎
	☐ urinary calculus; urolith	尿〔結〕石
	☐ urinary disturbance	排尿障害
	☐ urinary incontinence	尿失禁
	☐ urinary tract candidiasis	尿路カンジダ症
	☐ urinary tract infection (UTI)	尿路感染症
	☐ urolithiasis; urinary tract stone disease	尿路結石症

9 Diseases and Disorders of the Reproductive System 生殖系の疾患・障害

1. ☐ **amenorrhea** — 無月経
2. ☐ balanoposthitis — 亀頭包皮炎
3. ☐ **breast cancer** — 乳がん
4. ☐ **cervical cancer** — 子宮頚がん
5. ☐ **climacteric disturbance;** — 更年期障害；更年期症候群
6. **menopausal syndrome**
7. ☐ condyloma acuminatum — 尖圭コンジローム症
8. ☐ dysmenorrhea; menstruation — 月経困難症
9. disturbance; premenstrual
10. irregularity
11. ☐ endometriosis — 子宮内膜症
12. ☐ epididymitis — 副睾丸炎，精巣上体炎
13. ☐ epimenorrhea — 頻発月経
14. ☐ genital herpes; herpes genitals — 陰部ヘルペス
15. ☐ **gonorrhea** — **淋疾，淋病**
16. ☐ hematospermia — 血精液症
17. ☐ hydatidiform mole — 胞状奇体
18. ☐ **impotence; erectile dysfunction** — インポテンス，性交不能症；
19. **(ED)** — 勃起障害
20. ☐ leukorrhea; vaginal discharge — 帯下（こしけ）；おりもの
21. ☐ mastalgia — 乳房痛
22. ☐ mastitis — 乳腺炎，乳房炎
23. ☐ menorrhagia; menstrual pain — 生理痛
24. ☐ **menopause** — **閉経**
25. ☐ premature menopause; precocious — 早発閉経
26. menopause
27. ☐ menoxenia — 月経異常

1	☐ metrorrhagia	不正〔子宮〕出血
2	☐ oligomenorrhea	希発月経
3	☐ oophoritis	卵巣炎
4	☐ ovarian cancer	卵巣がん
5	☐ ovarian dysfunction	卵巣機能障害
6	☐ premenstrual syndrome (PMS);	月経前症候群；月経前緊張
7	premenstrual tension (PMT)	症
8	☐ salpingitis	卵管炎
9	☐ **sexually transmitted diseases**	**性感染症**
10	**(STD)**	
11	☐ Sheehan syndrome; postpartum	シーハン症候群；
12	hypopituitarism	分娩後下垂体機能低下症
13	☐ sperma invasion	精子侵襲症
14	☐ spermatic cord tortion	精索捻転症
15	☐ spermatocele	精液瘤
16	☐ testicular tumor	精巣（睾丸）腫瘍
17	☐ uterine myoma	子宮筋腫
18	☐ uterine rupture	子宮破裂
19	☐ uterine sarcoma	子宮肉腫

9-1. Pregnancy and Childbirth　　妊娠・出産

22	☐ **abortion**	**流産**
23	☐ abruptio placentae	〔常位〕胎盤早期剥離
24	☐ **birth weight**	**出生体重**
25	☐ extremely low birth weight (ELBW)	超低出生体重児；超未熟児
26	infant; extremely immature infant	
27	☐ low birth weight (LBW) infant;	低出生体重児；未熟児
28	immature infant	
29	☐ **childbirth**	**出産**
30	☐ **delivery**	**分娩**

Part 2 **Medical Terms** 医学・医療の基本英単語

1. ☐ **due date** 〔出産〕予定日
2. ☐ **fertilization** 受精
3. ☐ in vitro fertilization (IVF) 体外受精
4. ☐ **fetus**; fetal 胎児；胎児〔性〕の
5. ☐ **infant**; infantile 小児, 乳児；小児〔性〕の,
6. 乳児〔性〕の
7. ☐ **infertility** 不妊症, 不育症
8. ☐ **insemination** 授精
9. ☐ artificial insemination 人工授精
10. ☐ **labor** 分娩〔期〕, 陣痛
11. ☐ labor pains 陣痛
12. ☐ **maternity** 母性
13. ☐ maternity-blue syndrome マタニティブルー症候群
14. ☐ newborn; neonate; neonatal 新生児；新生児〔性〕の
15. ☐ **pregnancy**; gestation 妊娠《*adj.* pregnant》
16. ☐ ectopic pregnancy 子宮外妊娠
17. ☐ multiple pregnancy 多胎妊娠
18. ☐ rupture of membranes; 破水
19. amniorrhexis
20. ☐ premature rupture of membranes 早期破水
21. (PROM)
22. ☐ sterility 生殖不能, 不妊〔症〕

10 Diseases and Disorders of the Immune System 免疫系の疾患・障害

10-1. Systemic Autoimmune Diseases; Collagen Diseases 全身性自己免疫疾患;膠原病

- [ ] acquired immunodeficiency syndrome (AIDS); human immunodeficiency virus (HIV) infection — 後天性免疫不全症候群,エイズ;ヒト免疫不全ウイルス感染症
- [ ] adult-onset Still disease (AOSD) — 成人スティル病
- [ ] antiphospholipid antibody syndrome (APS) — 抗リン脂質抗体症候群
- [ ] eosinophilia-myalgia syndrome — 好酸球増加・筋痛症候群
- [ ] eosinophilic fasciitis; Shulman syndrome — 好酸球性筋膜炎;シュルマン(シャルマン)症候群
- [ ] Felty syndrome — フェルティ症候群
- [ ] human adjuvant disease — ヒト・アジュバント病
- [ ] lupus erythematosus — エリテマトーデス,紅斑性狼瘡
- [ ]   discoid lupus erythematosus (DLE) — 円板状エリテマトーデス
- [ ]   systemic lupus erythematosus (SLE) — 〔全身性〕エリテマトーデス
- [ ] mixed connective tissue disease (MCTD) — 混合性結合組織病
- [ ] Reiter syndrome (disease) — ライター症候群
- [ ] remitting seronegative symmetrical synovitis with pitting edema — RS3PE症候群
- [ ] sarcoidosis; Boeck disease — サルコイドーシス;ベック病
- [ ] seronegative spondyloarthropathy — 血清反応陰性脊椎炎
- [ ] Sjögren syndrome (SjS; SS) — シェーグレン症候群
- [ ] Wegener's granulomatosis (WG) — ウェゲナー肉芽腫症

10-2. Immunodeficiency Diseases (Disorders)　免疫不全症

- ☐ bare lymphocyte syndrome　　　　　不全リンパ球症候群
- ☐ chronic glanulomatous disease (CGD)　慢性肉芽腫症
- ☐ common variable immunodeficiency (CVID)　分類不能型免疫不全症
- ☐ familial Mediterranean fever; familial paroxysmal polyserositis　家族性地中海熱
- ☐ hyperimmunogloblin E syndrome　高IgE症候群
- ☐ **immunodeficiency**　**免疫不全症**
- ☐ severe combined immunodeficiency (SCID)　重症複合型免疫不全症
- ☐ X-linked combined immunodeficiency disease　X連鎖〔性〕複合免疫不全症

11 Endocrine, Nutritional and Metabolic Diseases
内分泌・栄養・代謝疾患

11-1. Endocrine Diseases and Disorders　内分泌疾患・障害

- [ ] acromegaly; acromegalic gigantism　　先端巨大症
- [ ] adrenal tumor　　副腎腫瘍
- [ ] adrenocortical hyperplasia　　副腎皮質過形成
- [ ] adrenocortical insufficiency　　副腎皮質不全(機能低下症)
- [ ] primary chronic adrenocortical insufficiency; Addison disease　　原発性(一次性)慢性副腎皮質不全(機能低下症);アジソン病
- [ ] adrenogenital syndrome (AGS)　　副腎性器症候群
- [ ] aldosteronism　　アルドステロン症
- [ ] primary aldosteronism; Conn syndrome; primary hyperlipidemia　　原発性アルドステロン症;コン症候群;原発性高脂血症
- [ ] secondary aldosteronism　　続発性アルドステロン症
- [ ] **amyloidosis**　　**アミロイドーシス**
- [ ] carcinoid syndrome　　カルチノイド症候群
- [ ] Cushing disease　　クッシング病
- [ ] **diabetes mellitus**　　**〔真性〕糖尿病**
- [ ] type 1 diabetes [mellitus]; insulin-dependent diabetes mellitus (IDDM)　　1型〔真性〕糖尿病;インスリン依存性糖尿病
- [ ] type 2 diabetes [mellitus]; non-insulin-dependent diabetes mellitus (NIDDM)　　2型〔真性〕糖尿病;インスリン非依存性糖尿病
- [ ] dwarfism　　低身長, 小人症
- [ ] dwarfism-immunopathy-asthma syndrome　　低身長・免疫障害・喘息症候群
- [ ] ectopic ACTH (adrenocorticotropic hormone) syndrome　　異所性ACTH(副腎皮質刺激ホルモン)症候群
- [ ] galactorrhea; lactorrhea　　乳〔汁〕漏〔出〕症

1	☐ gigantism; macrosomia; megasomia	巨人症
2	☐ pituitary gigantism	下垂体性巨人症
3	☐ glucocorticoid resistance syndrome	グルココルチコイド抵抗〔性〕症候群
5	☐ Hashimoto disease; Hashimoto thyroiditis; chronic thyroiditis	橋本病；橋本甲状腺炎；慢性甲状腺炎
7	☐ hyperparathyroidism	副甲状腺（上皮小体）機能亢進症
9	☐ hyperpituitarism	下垂体機能亢進症
10	☐ **hyperthyroidism**; Basedow disease; Graves disease	**甲状腺機能亢進症**；バセドウ病；グレーブズ病
12	☐ hypoparathyroidism	副甲状腺（上皮小体）機能低下症
14	☐ hypopituitarism	下垂体機能低下症
15	☐ hypothyroidism	甲状腺機能低下症
16	☐ inappropriate antidiuretic hormone (ADH) syndrome	抗利尿ホルモン（ADH）分泌異常症候群
18	☐ inappropriate prolactin syndrome	黄体刺激ホルモン（プロラクチン，PRL）分泌異常症候群
20	☐ ketoacidosis	ケトアシドーシス
21	☐ diabetic ketoacidosis (DKA)	糖尿病性ケトアシドーシス
22	☐ lysosomal disease	リソソーム（ライソゾーム）病
23	☐ masculinization	男性化《生理学的に男性の特徴．病理学的に両性の特徴を備えている。cf. virilism》
26	☐ nodular goiter; thyroid nodule	結節性甲状腺腫；甲状腺結節
27	☐ pheochromocytoma; chromaffin cell tumor	褐色細胞腫；クロム親和細胞腫
29	☐ polyendocrinopathy	多腺性内分泌不全症
30	☐ precocious puberty	思春期早発症

1. ☐ prolactin-producing adenoma　　プロラクチン産生腺腫
2. ☐ pseudohypoaldosteronism　　偽性低アルドステロン症
3. ☐ pseudohypoparathyroidism　　偽性副甲状腺機能低下症
4. ☐ resistance to thyroid hormone　　甲状腺ホルモン不応症
5. ☐ short stature　　小児の低身長
6. ☐ thyroid-stimulating hormone receptor disease　　甲状腺刺激ホルモン(TSH)受容体異常症
8. ☐ thyroid tumor　　甲状腺腫瘍
9. ☐ **thyroiditis**　　**甲状腺炎**
10. ☐ virilism　　男性化《女児，女性，思春期前の男性が，成熟した男性の身体的特徴を備えている。*cf.* masculinization》

11-2. Nutritional and Metabolic Diseases and Disorders　栄養・代謝疾患・障害

15. ☐ adiposity　　脂肪症
16. ☐ beriberi　　脚気
17. ☐ Bitot spot　　ビトー斑
18. ☐ dietary calcium deficiency　　食事性カルシウム欠乏症
19. ☐ dyslipidemia　　脂質異常症
20. ☐ emaciation; vitamin D deficiency　　るいそう；ビタミンD欠乏症
21. ☐ essential fatty acid deficiency　　必須脂肪酸欠乏症
22. ☐ folic acid deficiency　　葉酸欠乏症
23. ☐ **gout**　　**痛風**
24. ☐ hypercalcemia　　高カルシウム血症
25. ☐ **hypercholesterolemia**　　**高コレステロール血症**
26. ☐ hyperkalemia; hyperpotassemia　　高カリウム血症
27. ☐ **hyperlipidemia**　　**高脂血症**
28. ☐ hyperuricemia　　高尿酸血症
29. ☐ hypervitaminosis　　ビタミン過剰症
30. ☐ hypocalcemia　　低カルシウム血症

1	☐ hypokalemia; hypopotassemia	低カリウム血症
2	☐ hypoproteinemia	低たんぱく(蛋白)質血症
3	☐ iron deficiency	鉄欠乏症
4	☐ kwashiorkor	クワシオルコル
5	☐ lactose intolerance	乳糖不耐症
6	☐ Lesch-Nyhan syndrome (LNS);	レッシューナイハン症候群；
7	juvenile hyperuricemia syndrome	若年性高尿酸血症症候群
8	☐ **life style-related disease**	**生活習慣病**
9	☐ malabsorption syndrome	吸収不良症候群
10	☐ malnutrition	栄養失調，栄養欠乏症
11	☐ protein-energy malnutrition (PEM)	たんぱく(蛋白)質エネルギー
12		栄養障害
13	☐ marasmus	マラスマス，〔栄養性〕消耗症
14	☐ **metabolic syndrome**	**メタボリックシンドローム**
15	☐ moon face; cushingoid face	満月状(様)顔〔貌〕；クッシ
16		ング様顔貌
17	☐ mucopolysaccharidosis	ムコ多糖〔体蓄積〕症
18	☐ niacin deficiency; pellagra	ナイアシン欠乏症；ペラグラ
19	☐ nonalcoholic steatohepatitis (NASH);	非アルコール性脂肪肝
20	nonalcoholic fatty liver disease (NAFLD)	
21	☐ nutrition disorder	栄養疾患
22	☐ **obesity**	**肥満〔症〕**
23	☐ abdominal obesity	腹部肥満
24	☐ childhood obesity	小児肥満症
25	☐ simple obesity	単純肥満症《一次性/原発性の肥満》
26	☐ symptomatic obesity; secondary obesity	症候性肥満；二次性肥満
27	☐ obesity hypoventilation syndrome	肥満低換気症候群
28	☐ overnutrition	過栄養
29	☐ phenylketonuria	〔古典型〕フェニルケトン尿症
30	☐ potassium depletion	カリウム枯渇

1	☐ renal osteodystrophy	腎性骨ジストロフィー（異栄養症）
2		
3	☐ rickets; rachitis	くる病
4	☐ saccharometabolic disorder	糖質代謝異常
5	☐ scurvy; scorbutus; vitamin C deficiency	壊血病；ビタミンC欠乏症
6		
7	☐ slim disease	やせ病
8	☐ thiamin deficiency	チアミン欠乏症
9	☐ uric acid metabolic disorder	尿酸代謝異常
10	☐ vitamin A (B; C; D; E; K) deficiency	ビタミンA（B；C；D；E；K）欠乏症

12 Hematopoietic Diseases
造血系疾患

1. ☐ agammaglobulinemia — 無ガンマグロブリン血症
2. ☐ X-linked agammaglobulinemia (XLA) — X連鎖性無ガンマグロブリン血症
3. ☐ **anemia** — **貧血**
4. ☐ aplastic anemia — 再生不良性貧血
5. ☐ bleeding anemia — 出血性貧血
6. ☐ hemolytic anemia — 溶血性貧血
7. ☐ iron deficiency anemia (IDA) — 鉄欠乏性貧血
8. ☐ Mediterranean anemia; thalassemia — 地中海貧血；サラセミア
9. ☐ megaloblastic anemia — 巨赤芽球性貧血
10. ☐ pernicious anemia — 悪性貧血
11. ☐ sickle cell disease (SCD); sickle cell anemia — 鎌状赤血球症；鎌状赤血球貧血
12. ☐ vitamin B_{12} deficiency anemia — ビタミンB_{12}欠乏性貧血
13. ☐ Banti syndrome — バンティ症候群
14. ☐ Castleman disease; mediastinal giant lymph node hyperplasia — キャッスルマン病；縦隔巨大リンパ節過形成
15. ☐ elephantiasis — 象皮病
16. ☐ erythrocytosis — 赤血球増加症
17. ☐ familial erythrocytosis — 家族性赤血球増加症
18. ☐ heavy chain disease — 重鎖病
19. ☐ hemoglobinemia — 血色素尿症，ヘモグロビン血症
20. ☐ paroxysmal nocturnal hemoglobinemia (PNH) — 発作性夜間血色素尿症
21. ☐ **hemophilia** — **血友病**
22. ☐ histiocytosis — 組織球増殖症
23. ☐ **leukemia** — **白血病**

1	☐ acute lymphocytic (lymphatic) leukemia (ALL)	急性リンパ性白血病
3	☐ acute monocytic leukemia (AMoL)	急性単球性白血病
4	☐ acute myeloid (myelogenous) leukemia (AML)	急性骨髄性白血病
6	☐ adult T-cell leukemia/lymphoma (ATL)	成人型T細胞白血病／リンパ腫
7	☐ chronic lymphocytic (lymphatic) leukemia (CLL)	慢性リンパ性白血病
9	☐ chronic myelocytic (myelogenous) leukemia (CML)	慢性骨髄性白血病
11	☐ leukemoid reaction	類白血病反応
12	☐ leukocytosis	白血球増多症
13	☐ leukopenia	白血球減少症
14	☐ lymph node tuberculosis	リンパ節結核
15	**☐ lymphadenitis**	**リンパ節炎**
16	☐ abscess forming reticular lymphadenitis; cat scratch disease	化膿性肉芽腫性リンパ節炎；猫ひっかき病
18	☐ histiocytic necrotizing lymphadenitis	組織球性壊死性リンパ節炎，亜急性壊死性リンパ節炎，菊池病
20	☐ nonspecific lymphadenitis	非特異性リンパ節炎
21	☐ toxoplasmic lymphadenitits	トキソプラスマ性リンパ節炎
22	☐ tuberculous lymphadenitis	結核性リンパ節炎
23	**☐ lymphadenopathy**	**リンパ節症**
24	☐ dermatopathic lymphadenopathy	皮膚病性リンパ節症
25	☐ drug-induced lymphadenopathy	薬剤性リンパ節症
26	☐ immunoblastic lymphadenopathy (IBL)	免疫芽球性リンパ節症
27	☐ lymphangiectasis	リンパ管拡張症
28	☐ lymphangitis	リンパ管炎
29	☐ lymphatic abnormality	リンパ管異常
30	☐ lymphedema	リンパ浮腫

☐	lymphocele	リンパ嚢腫
☐	lymphohistiocytosis	リンパ組織球増多症
☐	familial hemophagocytic lymphohistiocytosis (FHL)	家族性血球貪食リンパ組織球増多症症候群
☐	**lymphoma**	**リンパ腫**
☐	Burkitt lymphoma	バーキットリンパ腫
☐	diffuse large B-cell lymphoma	びまん性大細胞型B細胞性リンパ腫
☐	follicular lymphoma	濾胞性リンパ腫
☐	Hodgkin lymphoma	ホジキンリンパ腫
☐	lymphoblastic lymphoma	リンパ芽球性リンパ腫
☐	malignant lymphoma (ML)	悪性リンパ腫
☐	marginal zone lymphoma	辺縁層リンパ腫
☐	peripheral T-cell lymphoma	末梢性T細胞性リンパ腫
☐	lymphoproliferative syndrome	リンパ増殖症候群
☐	autoimmune lymphoproliferative syndrome (ALPS)	自己免疫性リンパ増殖症候群
☐	lymphosarcoma	リンパ肉腫
☐	macroglobulinemia	マクログロブリン血症
☐	primary macroglobulinemia; Waldenström macroglobulinemia	原発性マクログロブリン血症；ヴァルデンストレームマクログロブリン血症
☐	mononucleosis	単核球症
☐	mycosis fungoides	菌状息肉腫
☐	**myelodysplastic syndrome (MDS)**	**骨髄異形成症候群**
☐	myelofibrosis	骨髄線維症
☐	**myeloma**	**骨髄腫**
☐	endothelial myeloma; Ewing sarcoma	内皮性骨髄腫；ユーイング肉腫
☐	multiple myeloma	多発性骨髄腫
☐	myeloproliferative disorders (MPD)	骨髄増殖疾患群
☐	neutropenia	好中球減少症

1	☐ polycythemia vera	真性赤血球増加症
2	☐ **purpura**	**紫斑〔病〕**
3	☐ idiopathic thrombocytopenic purpura (ITP)	特発性血小板減少性紫斑病
4	☐ thrombotic thrombocytopenic purpura (TTP)	血栓性血小板減少性紫斑病
6	☐ Sézary syndrome	セザリー症候群
7	☐ thrombocythemia	血小板血症
8	☐ **thrombocytopenia**	**血小板減少症**
9	☐ thymus hyperplasia	胸腺過形成
10	☐ von Willebrand syndrome	フォン・ヴィルブランド病

13 Congenital and Hereditary Diseases and Disorders　先天性/遺伝性の疾患・障害

- [ ] adenosine deaminase (ADA) deficiency　アデノシンデアミナーゼ（ADA）欠損症
- [ ] adrenal enzyme deficiency　副腎酵素欠損症
- [ ] Aicardi syndrome　アイカルディ症候群
- [ ] albinism　白皮症
- [ ] Angelman syndrome (AS)　アンジェルマン症候群
- [ ] anhidrotic ectodermal dysplasia (AED)　無汗性外胚葉形成異常症
- [ ] aniridia　無虹彩
- [ ] Apert syndrome; acrocephalopolysyndactyly　アペール症候群；尖頭合指〔症〕
- [ ] aproctia; anal atresia; proctaresia　鎖肛症
- [ ] biopterin metabolic disorder　ビオプテリン代謝異常症
- [ ] CATCH22 syndrome; DiGeorge syndrome　キャッチ22症候群；ディジョージ症候群《Cardiac anomaly 心血管異常; Abnormal facies 異常顔貌; Thymic hypoplasia 胸腺低形成; Cleft palate 口蓋裂; Hypocalcemia 低カルシウム血症》
- [ ] CHARGE association [syndrome]　チャージ連合［症候群］《Coloboma 眼の一部欠損; Heart disease 心疾患; Atresia choanae 後鼻腔閉鎖; Retarded growth and development and/or CNS anomalies 成長発育遅滞および/または中枢神経系の奇形; Genital hyperplasia 性器発育不全; Ear anomalies and/or deafness 聴力異常および/または聾》

1	☐ cleft lip and palate	口蓋裂
2	☐ chromosomal syndrome	染色体症候群
3	☐ congenital adrenal hyperplasia (CHA)	先天性副腎皮質過形成
4	☐ congenital defects	先天性欠損症
5	☐ congenital heart disease	先天性心疾患
6	☐ congenital hydronephrosis	先天性水腎症
7	☐ congenital insensitivity to pain with anhidrosis (CIPA)	先天性無痛無汗症
9	☐ congenital photomyoclonus; de Lange syndrome	遺伝性光ミオクローヌス ド・ランゲ症候群
11	☐ Crigler-Najjar syndrome	クリグラー－ナジャー症候群
12	☐ cystic fibrosis (CF)	嚢胞性線維症
13	☐ Down syndrome	ダウン症候群
14	☐ ectopic testis	異所性精巣(睾丸)
15	☐ Edwards syndrome; trisomy 18 syndrome	エドワーズ症候群；18トリソミー症候群
17	☐ epidermolysis bullosa hereditaria	先天性表皮水疱症
18	☐ familial polyposis coli (FPC)	家族性大腸ポリポーシス
19	☐ fibrodysplasia ossificans progressiva	進行性骨化性線維異形成症
20	☐ fragile X syndrome	脆弱X症候群，フラジャイルエックス症候群
22	☐ glycogenosis	糖原病
23	☐ heredoataxia	遺伝性運動失調〔症〕
24	☐ heterotaxia; visceral inversion	内臓逆位症
25	☐ hermaphroditism	半陰陽
26	☐ Hischsprung disease; congenital megacolon	ヒルシュスプルング病；先天性巨大結腸
28	☐ homocystinuria	ホモシスチン尿症
29	☐ hydrocephalus	水頭症
30	☐ Janus kinase 3 defect	ヤヌスキナーゼ3欠損症

☐	levocardia; sinistrocardia	右胸心；右心症
☐	malformation syndrome	奇形症候群
☐	maple syrup urine disease	メープルシロップ尿症
☐	Meckel-Gruber syndrome	メッケル-グルーバー症候群
☐	megalencephaly	巨大脳髄腫
☐	Miller-Dieker syndrome; lissencephaly	ミラー-ディッカー症候群；滑脳症
☐	monilethrix; beaded hair	連珠毛
☐	neurofibromatosis type 1 (NF1); von Recklinghausen disease	神経線維腫症1型；フォン・レックリングハウゼン病
☐	neurofibromatosis type 2 (NF2)	神経線維腫症2型
☐	Patau syndrome; trisomy 13 syndrome	パトー症候群；13トリソミー症候群
☐	Prader-Willi syndrome (PWS)	プラダー-ウィリー症候群
☐	phacomatosis	母斑症
☐	phocomelia	アザラシ肢症
☐	polydactyly	多指症
☐	progeria	早老症
☐	Rubinstein-Taybi syndrome	ルビンスタイン-テイビー（タイビー）症候群
☐	spina bifida	二分脊椎
☐	Turner syndrome; XO syndrome	ターナー症候群；XO症候群
☐	velocardiofacial syndrome	口蓋心顔面症候群
☐	Williams syndrome (WS); elfin facies syndrome	ウィリアムズ症候群；妖精様顔〔貌〕症候群
☐	Wilson disease	ウィルソン病
☐	Wiskott-Aldrich syndrome (WAS)	ウィスコット-アルドリッチ症候群

14 Mental Health Diseases and Disorders
心因性・精神疾患と障害

1	☐ acute stress disorder (ASD)	急性ストレス障害
2	☐ adjustment disorder	適応障害
3	☐ affective disorder; emotional disorder	感情障害；情動障害
5	☐ agoraphobia	広場恐怖〔症〕
6	☐ **alcoholism**	**アルコール依存症**
7	☐ **amnesia**	**健忘〔症〕**
8	☐ dissociative amnesia; dissociative fugue	解離性健忘〔症〕；解離性遁走
9	☐ transient global amnesia (TGA)	一過性全健忘〔症〕
10	☐ **anorexia**	**食欲不振**
11	☐ anorexia nervosa (AN)	神経性食思不振症, 神経性無食欲症
13	☐ anxiety disorder	不安障害
14	☐ generalized anxiety disorder (GAD)	全般性不安障害
15	☐ separation anxiety disorder	分離不安障害
16	☐ Asperger syndrome	アスペルガー症候群, 高機能自閉症
18	☐ **attention-deficit/hyperactivity disorder (ADHD)**	**注意欠陥/多動性障害**
20	☐ **autism**	**自閉症**
21	☐ body dysmorphic disorder	身体醜形障害
22	☐ bulimia nervosa (BN)	神経性大食症
23	☐ burnout syndrome	バーンアウト〔シンドローム〕, 燃え尽き症候群
25	☐ catatonia	緊張性昏迷
26	☐ cognitive disorder	認知障害
27	☐ conduct disorder (CD)	行為障害

#	English	日本語
1	conversion disorder	転換性障害
2	**delirium**	**せん妄**
3	night delirium	夜間せん妄
4	**delusion**	**妄想**
5	[persistent] delusional disorder	〔持続性〕妄想性障害
6	**dementia**	**認知症**
7	Alzheimer dementia	アルツハイマー型認知症
8	depersonalization disorder	離人症障害
9	**depression**	**うつ(鬱)病, 抑うつ〔症〕**
10	geriatric depression	老年期うつ病
11	depressive state	抑うつ状態
12-13	**developmental disability/ disorder (DD)**	**発達障害**
14	pervasive developmental disorder (PDD)	広汎〔性〕発達障害
15	dissociative disorder	解離性障害
16	drug dependence	薬物依存
17	dysthymic disorder	気分変調性障害
18	eating disorder	摂食障害
19	**epilepsy**	**てんかん**
20	myochronic epilepsy	ミオクローヌス性てんかん
21	euphoria	多幸症
22	**hallucination**	**幻覚**
23	auditory hallucination	幻聴
24	visual hallucination	幻視
25	heterosexuality	異性愛
26	homosexuality	同性愛
27	hyperkinetic disorder	多動性障害
28	hypochondriasis; hypochondria	心気症；ヒポコンドリー〔症〕
29	identity disorder	同一性障害
30	dissociative identity disorder	解離性同一性障害

1	☐ gender identity disorder (GID)	性同一性障害
2	☐ intellectual impairment	知的障害
3	☐ **learning disability (LD)**	**学習障害**
4	☐ macropsia	大視症
5	☐ **mania**	**躁病**
6	☐ **manic-depressive disorder (psychosis); bipolar disorder**	**躁うつ病；双極性障害**
8	☐ **mental retardation (MR)**	**精神遅滞**
9	☐ micropsia	小視症
10	☐ mood disorder	気分障害
11	☐ mutism	無言症，緘黙（かんもく）症
12	☐ selective mutism	選択性緘黙〔症〕
13	☐ **neurosis**	**神経症**
14	☐ traumatic neurosis	外傷性神経症
15	☐ night terrors	睡眠時驚愕症，夜驚症
16	☐ obsessive-compulsive disorder (OCD)	強迫性障害
18	☐ oppositional defiant disorder (ODD)	反抗挑戦性障害
19	☐ pain disorder	疼痛性障害
20	☐ **panic disorder (PD)**	**パニック障害**
21	☐ paraphasia	錯語〔症〕
22	☐ pathological gambling	病的賭博
23	☐ pedophilia	小児性愛
24	☐ **personality disorder**	**人格障害**
25	☐ affective personality disorder	感情性人格障害
26	☐ antisocial personality disorder	反社会性人格障害
27	☐ asthenic personality disorder	無力性人格障害
28	☐ avoidant personality disorder	回避性人格障害
29	☐ borderline personality disorder	境界性人格障害
30	☐ cycloid personality disorder	循環性人格障害

1	☐ dependent personality disorder	依存性人格障害
2	☐ histrionic personality disorder;	演技性人格障害；ヒステリー
3	hysteric personality disorder	性人格障害
4	☐ narcissistic personality disorder	自己愛性人格障害
5	☐ obsessive-compulsive personality	強迫性人格障害
6	disorder	
7	☐ paranoid personality disorder	妄想性人格障害
8	☐ **phobia**	**恐怖〔症〕**
9	☐ pica	異食〔症〕
10	☐ polyphagia; hyperphagia	過食〔症〕
11	☐ **posttraumatic stress disorder**	**心的外傷後ストレス障害**
12	**(PTSD)**	
13	☐ **psychosis**	**精神病**
14	☐ hallucinatory psychosis	幻覚性精神病
15	☐ induced psychosis	感応精神病
16	☐ organic psychosis	器質性精神病
17	☐ postpartum psychosis	産後精神病
18	☐ symptomatic psychosis; organic	症候性精神障害；器質性精神
19	psychosis	病
20	☐ toxic psychosis	中毒性精神病
21	☐ **psychosomatic disorder (PSD)**	**心身症**
22	☐ REM sleep behavior disorder	レム睡眠行動障害
23	☐ Rett syndrome	レット症候群
24	☐ sadomasochism	サドマゾヒズム
25	☐ savant syndrome	サヴァン症候群
26	☐ schizoaffective disorder	統合失調感情障害
27	☐ **schizophrenia**	**統合失調症**
28	☐ schizophreniform disorder	統合失調症様障害
29	☐ schizotypal disorder	統合失調型障害
30	☐ sexual deviation	性〔的〕倒錯〔症〕

- ☐ shared psychotic disorder; 共有性精神病性障害
  folie à deux《仏》
- ☐ **sleep disorder; insomnia;** **睡眠障害；不眠〔症〕**
  sleeplessness
- ☐ somatization disorder 身体化障害
- ☐ somatoform disorder 身体表現性障害

> **COLUMN 接尾辞でわかる精神医学と心理学の違い**
>
> 　専門英語は，言葉の語尾から違いを見分けることができる。例えば，psychiatryとpsychologyは，-iatroが医師(ギリシャ語：iatros)，-logyは学問を意味するので，前者が精神医学，後者が心理学である。同様にgeriatrics(老人医学)とgerontology(老人学)も区別できる。
>
> 　因みに，-logyは，logos(言葉)に由来し，多くの学問の名称の語尾に付されている。聖書に「初めに言葉(logos)があった」と記されているように，言葉は強い力をもつものであった。さらにギリシャ時代に「理性・議論」の意味となり，理性に則って議論する学問が成立してきた。医学も例外ではなく，physiology(生理学)，cytology(細胞学)，hematology(血液学)，pathology(病理学)，immunology(免疫学)，otolaryngology(耳鼻咽喉科学)，urology(泌尿器科学)というように，-logyが付されている。
>
> 　ところで，psychiatryとpsychologyのpsych-は，ギリシャ神話に登場する美少女，プシュケ(Psychè＝人間の魂)に由来する。恋の神エロスErosと恋をした彼女に，エロスの母である愛と美の女神アフロディテは，プシュケに「冥界にある美の薬をもらってくれば許そう」と艱難を強いた。その宿題？を果たして，プシュケ(魂)とエロス(性愛)はようやく結婚できた，というBack to the future的お話しである。

15 Infectious Diseases
感染症

1. ☐ acariasis; acarinosis — ダニ刺症
2. ☐ anthrax — 炭疽
3. ☐ bacterial food poisoning — 細菌性食中毒
4. ☐ botulism — ボツリヌス症
5. ☐ bovine spongiform encephalopathy (BSE) — 牛海綿状脳症, 狂牛病
7. ☐ candidiasis — カンジダ症
8. ☐ **cholera** — **コレラ**
9. ☐ congenital cytomegalovirus (CMV) infection — 先天性サイトメガロウイルス感染症
11. ☐ coronavirus disease 2019 (COVID-19) — 新型コロナウイルス感染症
13. ☐ dengue fever — デング熱
14. ☐ diphtheria — ジフテリア
15. ☐ **dysentery** — **赤痢**
16. ☐ enterobiasis; oxyuriasis — 蟯虫症
17. ☐ epidemic parotiditis (parotitis); mumps — 流行性耳下腺炎; おたふくかぜ
19. ☐ erysipelas — 丹毒
20. ☐ foot-and-mouth disease (FMD) — 口蹄病
21. ☐ hand-foot-and-mouth disease (HFMD) — 手足口病
22. ☐ Hansen disease — ハンセン病
23. ☐ hemorrhagic fever — 出血熱
24. ☐ Ebola hemorrhagic fever — エボラ出血熱
25. ☐ herpes simplex; herpes labials; cold sore; fever blister — 単純ヘルペス；口唇ヘルペス
27. ☐ herpes zoster; shingles; zona — 帯状疱疹（ヘルペス）

1	☐ hospital-acquired infection;	院内感染
2	nosocominal infection	
3	**influenza; flu; grippe**	**インフルエンザ**
4	☐ avian influenza	トリインフルエンザ
5	☐ H1N1 influenza	H1N1インフルエンザ
6	☐ new strain of [pandemic] influenza	新型インフルエンザ
7	☐ neonatal toxic-shock-syndrome-like	新生児TSS様発疹症
8	exanthematous disease (NTED)	
9	☐ nontuberculous mycobacterial	非結核性抗酸菌症
10	disease	
11	☐ paratyphoid fever	パラチフス
12	☐ pediculosis	シラミ症
13	☐ pertussis; whooping cough	百日咳
14	☐ pharyngoconjunctival fever (PCF)	咽頭結膜熱，プール熱
15	☐ **rabies**	**狂犬病**
16	☐ rheumatic fever	リウマチ熱
17	☐ **rubella**	**風疹，三日はしか**
18	☐ **rubeola; measles**	**麻疹，はしか**
19	☐ scarlet fever	猩紅熱
20	☐ **sepsis**	**敗血症**
21	☐ smallpox	天然痘，疱瘡
22	☐ syphilis	梅毒
23	☐ **tetanus**	**破傷風**
24	☐ toxic shock syndrome (TSS)	〔中〕毒性ショック症候群
25	☐ toxoplasmosis	トキソプラズマ症
26	☐ trachoma	トラコーマ
27	☐ trichomoniasis	トリコモナス症
28	☐ trichomoniasis vaginalis	腟トリコモナス症
29	☐ typhoid fever	腸チフス
30	☐ typhus	チフス

1	☐ epidemic typhus	発疹チフス
2	☐ **varicella**; **chickenpox**	水痘；水ぼうそう

15-1. Pathogenic organisms　　病原微生物

5	☐ **ameba**; **amebic**	アメーバ〔の〕
6	☐ Bacillus anthracis	炭疽菌
7	☐ **bacterium**; **bactrial**; **germ**	細菌；細菌の；バイキン
8	☐ drug-resistant bacteria	薬剤耐性菌
9	☐ botulinum	ボツリヌス菌
10	☐ candida	カンジダ
11	☐ chlamydia; chlamydial	クラミジア〔の〕
12	☐ coccus; coccal	球菌《*pl.* cocci》
13	☐ enterobacterium	腸内細菌
14	☐ **Escherichia coli**	**大腸菌**
15	☐ enterohemorrhagic Escherichia coli (EHEC)	腸管出血性大腸菌
17	☐ **fungus**	真菌《*pl.* fungi》
18	☐ **parasite**	寄生生物，寄生虫
19	☐ protozoan	原虫
20	☐ rickettsia	リケッチア
21	☐ salmonella	サルモネラ菌
22	☐ **staphylococcus**; **staphylococcal**	ブドウ球菌〔の〕
23	☐ **Staphylococcus aureus**	**黄色ブドウ球菌**
24	☐ methicillin-resistant Staphylococcus aureus (MRSA)	メチシリン耐性黄色ブドウ球菌
26	☐ **streptococcus**; **streptococcal**	**連鎖球菌**〔の〕
27	☐ **Streptococcus pneumoniae**	**肺炎連鎖球菌**
28	☐ toxoplasma	トキソプラズマ
29	☐ **virus**; **viral**	ウイルス〔の〕
30	☐ cytomegalovirus (CMV)	サイトメガロウイルス

1. ☐ dengue virus — デング熱ウイルス
2. ☐ Ebola virus — エボラウイルス
3. ☐ Epstein–Barr virus (EBV) — エプスタイン−バーウイルス
4. ☐ herpes simplex virus (HSV) — 単純ヘルペスウイルス
5. ☐ human immunodeficiency virus (HIV) — ヒト免疫不全ウイルス
6. ☐ human papillomavirus (HPV) — ヒト乳頭腫ウイルス
7. ☐ norovirus — ノロウイルス

COLUMN 接頭辞で変わる感染症の規模

人々を不安にさせる感染症 infectious diseaseは, endemic, epidemic, pandemicと, 接頭辞の違いで流行の規模の拡大が表される。endemic(風土病, 地方病)は, 接頭辞en-(中に)＋demic(demos: 人々) ＋ ic(形容詞語尾)と, 読んで字のごとく, 限定された地域で流行する。同様に, epidemic(流行病)は, epi-(among: 間に)が「人々の間に広く広まる」を示し, さらにpandemicは, pan-(全〜, 総〜)によって, 「世界的(全国的)に広がる流行病」となる。

記憶に新しいpandemic と言えば, 2009年に豚インフルエンザ(swine flu)*が流行, 世界規模で拡大した。豚の組織にあるウイルスが人へ感染するもので, WHOは病気の広がりをepidemicからpandemicへと変更し, 対策を講じた。

因みにinfectiousは, 病気に限らず, 癖や感情, 言葉遣いなども「人に移りやすい」という意味もある。Her happy face is infectious.と言われたいものだ。

Notes: swine flluという名称は, 宗教的にも, また畜産に従事する人々に対しても問題があるために, 現在では, influenza A (H1N1)(日本では「新型インフルエンザA」)と呼ばれている。

Part 3

Terms of Body Parts and Functions

人体各部の名称と機能の英単語

1 Head and Neck
頭頸部

1. □ cheek — 頬
2. □ chin; mentum — 顎の先：おとがい（頤）
3. □ forehead — 額
4. □ head — 頭
5. □ jaw — 顎
6. □ lower jaw; mandible; mandibular — 下顎；下顎骨；下顎〔骨〕の
7. □ upper jaw; maxilla; maxillary — 上顎；上顎骨；上顎〔骨〕の
8. □ nape — うなじ（項）
9. □ neck; cervix; cervical — 首；頚〔部〕；頚〔部〕の
10. □ parathyroid gland — 副甲状腺
11. □ temple; temporal — 側頭，こめかみ：側頭の，
12. こめかみの
13. □ thyroid gland — 甲状腺

1-1. Bones, Ligaments and Joints　骨・靭帯・関節

16. □ alveolar arch — 歯槽弓
17. □ alveolar process — 歯槽突起
18. □ anterior clinoid process — 前床突起
19. □ atlas — 環椎，第1頚椎
20. □ axis — 軸椎，第2頚椎
21. □ carotid tubercle — 頚動脈結節，第6頚椎
22. □ cervical vertebrae — 頚椎
23. □ dental alveolus — 歯槽
24. □ ethmoid [bone] — 篩骨
25. □ ethmoidal labyrinth — 篩骨迷路
26. □ external acoustic (auditory) pore — 外耳孔
27. □ foramen magnum — 大〔後頭〕孔

Part 3 **Terms of Body Parts and Functions**　人体各部の名称と機能の英単語

1	☐ foramen ovale	卵円孔
2	☐ frontal bone	前頭骨
3	☐ glabella	眉間
4	☐ hyoid bone	舌骨
5	☐ **incus**	**キヌタ（砧）骨**
6	☐ internal acoustic opening	内耳孔
7	☐ lacrimal bone	涙骨
8	☐ **malleus**	**ツチ（槌）骨**
9	☐ mastoid process	乳様突起
10	☐ middle nasal concha	中鼻甲介
11	☐ nasal crest	鼻稜
12	☐ occipital bone	後頭骨
13	☐ **orbit**; orbital	**眼窩**；眼窩の
14	☐ orbital process	眼窩突起
15	☐ palatine bone	口蓋骨
16	☐ parietal bone	頭頂骨
17	☐ pyramidal process	錐体突起
18	☐ sella turcica	トルコ鞍
19	☐ **skull**	**頭蓋**
20	☐ sphenoid [bone]	蝶形骨
21	☐ **stapes**	**アブミ（鐙）骨**
22	☐ temporal bone	側頭骨
23	☐ vertebra prominens	隆椎，第 7 頸椎
24	☐ zygomatic bone	頬骨

1-2. Muscles　　　　　　　　　　　　筋肉

27	☐ buccinator [muscle]	頬筋
28	☐ cricothyroid [muscle]	輪状甲状筋
29	☐ depressor anguli oris [muscle]	口角下制筋
30	☐ epicranius [muscle]	頭蓋表筋

1	☐ extraocular muscles; ocular muscles	外眼筋；眼筋
2	☐ frontalis [muscle]	前頭筋
3	☐ genioglossus [muscle]	おとがい舌筋
4	☐ geniohyoid [muscle]	おとがい舌骨筋
5	☐ inferior constrictor [muscle] of pharynx	下咽頭収縮筋
7	☐ lateral pterygoid [muscle]	外側翼突筋
8	☐ lateral rectus [muscle]	外側直筋
9	☐ levator anguli oris [muscle]	口角挙筋
10	☐ longissimus cervicis [muscle]	頚最長筋
11	☐ longus capitis [muscle]	頭長筋
12	☐ longus colli [muscle]	頚長筋
13	☐ masseter [muscle]	咬筋
14	☐ medial pterygoid [muscle]	内側翼突筋
15	☐ medial rectus [muscle]	内側直筋
16	☐ mentalis [muscle]	おとがい筋
17	☐ middle constrictor [muscle] of pharynx	中咽頭収縮筋
19	☐ nasalis [muscle]	鼻筋
20	☐ occipitalis [muscle]	後頭筋
21	☐ occipitofrontalis [muscle]	後頭前頭筋
22	☐ orbicularis oculi [muscle]	眼輪筋
23	☐ orbicularis oris [muscle]	口輪筋
24	☐ procerus [muscle]	鼻根筋
25	☐ risorius [muscle]	笑筋
26	☐ scalenus anterior muscle	前斜角筋
27	☐ superior pharyngeal constrictor [muscle]	上咽頭収縮筋
29	☐ temporalis [muscle]	側頭筋
30	☐ temporoparietalis [muscle]	側頭頭頂筋

Part 3 **Terms of Body Parts and Functions** 人体各部の名称と機能の英単語

☐ zygomaticus major [muscle]	大頬骨筋
☐ zygomaticus minor [muscle]	小頬骨筋

1-3. Nerves 神経

- ☐ abducent nerve (CN VI) 外転神経《第6脳神経》
- ☐ accessory nerve (CN XI) 副神経《第11脳神経》
- ☐ **central nerve** **中枢神経**
- ☐   central nervous system (CNS) 中枢神経系
- ☐ cervical nerve 頚神経
- ☐ cochlear nerve; auditory nerve 蝸牛神経；聴神経
- ☐ cranial nerves (CN) 脳神経
- ☐ epipharyngeal nerve 上咽頭神経
- ☐ **facial nerve (CN VII)** **顔面神経**《第7脳神経》
- ☐ glossopharyngeal nerve (CN IX) 舌咽神経《第9脳神経》
- ☐ hypoglossal nerve (CN XII) 舌下神経《第12脳神経》
- ☐ oculomotor nerve (CN III) 動眼神経《第3脳神経》
- ☐ **olfactory nerve (CN I)** **嗅神経**《第1脳神経》
- ☐ **optic nerve (CN II)** **視神経**《第2脳神経》
- ☐ supraorbital nerve 眼窩上神経
- ☐ terminal nerve 終神経
- ☐ trigeminal nerve (CN V) 三叉神経《第5脳神経》
- ☐ trochlear nerve (CN IV) 滑車神経《第4脳神経》
- ☐ vagus nerve (CN X) 迷走神経《第10脳神経》
- ☐ vestibular nerve 前庭神経
- ☐ vestibulocochlear nerve (CN VIII) 内耳神経《第8脳神経》
- ☐ zygomatic nerve 頬骨神経

1-4. Blood Vessels 血管

- [ ] basal vein — 脳底静脈
- [ ] **carotid arteries** — **頚動脈**
  - [ ] common carotid artery — 総頚動脈
  - [ ] external carotid artery — 外頚動脈
  - [ ] internal carotid artery — 内頚動脈
- [ ] cerebellar arteries — 小脳の動脈
  - [ ] anterior inferior cerebellar artery — 前下小脳動脈
  - [ ] posterior inferior cerebellar artery — 後下小脳動脈
  - [ ] superior cerebellar artery — 上小脳動脈
- [ ] cerebral arteries — 大脳の動脈
  - [ ] anterior cerebral artery — 前大脳動脈
  - [ ] middle cerebral artery — 中大脳動脈
  - [ ] posterior cerebral artery — 後大脳動脈
- [ ] cerebral veins — 大脳の静脈
  - [ ] anterior cerebral vein — 前大脳静脈
  - [ ] deep middle cerebral vein — 深中大脳静脈
  - [ ] great cerebral vein — 大大脳静脈
  - [ ] superficial middle cerebral vein — 浅中大脳静脈
- [ ] communicating arteries — 交通動脈
  - [ ] anterior communicating artery — 前交通動脈
  - [ ] posterior communicating artery — 後交通動脈
- [ ] **jugular veins** — **頚静脈**
  - [ ] external jugular vein — 外頚静脈
  - [ ] internal jugular vein — 内頚静脈
- [ ] ophthalmic artery — 眼動脈
- [ ] retinal artery — 網膜動脈
- [ ] retinal vein — 網膜静脈
- [ ] vertebral artery — 椎骨動脈
- [ ] vestibular aqueduct — 前庭水管

1-5. Brain 脳

- **arachnoid [mater]** クモ膜
- **area** 野
  - association area 連合野
  - Brodmann areas ブロードマン野
  - cortical area 皮質野
  - primary motor area 一次運動野
  - sensorial (sensory) areas 感覚野, 知覚野
  - sensorimotor area 感覚運動野
- association fiber 連合線維
- basal ganglia 大脳基底核
- **blood brain barrier (BBB)** 血液脳関門
- **brainstem** 脳幹
  - reticular formation of brainstem 脳幹網様体
- **center** 中枢
  - expiratory center 呼息中枢
  - inspiratory center 吸息中枢
  - motor speech center; Broca center (area) 運動性言語中枢;ブローカ中枢(野)
  - respiratory center 呼吸中枢
  - sensory center 感覚中枢
  - sensory speech center; Wernicke center (area) 感覚性言語中枢;ウェルニッケ中枢(野)
  - speech center 言語中枢
  - swallowing center 嚥下中枢
  - yawning center あくび中枢
- **cortex** 皮質
  - association cortex 連合皮質
  - auditory cortex (area) 聴覚皮質(野)
  - cerebellar cortex 小脳皮質
  - cerebral cortex 大脳皮質

1	☐ frontal cortex (area)	前頭皮質（野）
2	☐ motor cortex	運動皮質
3	☐ premotor cortex (area)	運動前皮質（野）
4	☐ sensory cortex	感覚皮質
5	☐ visual cortex (area)	視覚皮質（野）
6	☐ **cerebellum; cerebellar**	**小脳；小脳の**
7	☐ **cerebrum; cerebral**	**大脳；大脳の**
8	☐ **cervical [spinal] cord**	**頚部脊髄，頚髄**
9	☐ **corpus callosum**	**脳梁**
10	☐ splenium of corpus callosum	脳梁膨大部
11	☐ corticobulbar tract	皮質延髄路
12	☐ corticospinal tract	皮質脊髄路
13	☐ dentatum	歯状核
14	☐ **dura [mater]**	**硬膜**
15	☐ extrapyramidal [motor] system	錐体外路〔運動〕系
16	☐ gray matter	灰白質
17	☐ **hemisphere**	**半球**
18	☐ cerebellar hemisphere	小脳半球
19	☐ cerebral hemisphere	大脳半球
20	☐ **hippocampus**; hippocampal	**海馬**；海馬の
21	☐ **hypophysis; pituitary gland**	**下垂体**
22	☐ **hypothalamus**; hypothalamic	**視床下部**；視床下部の
23	☐ laryngeal prominence; Adam's apple	喉頭隆起；喉仏
24	☐ limbic system	〔大脳〕辺縁系
25	☐ **lobe**	**葉**
26	☐ frontal lobe	前頭葉
27	☐ occipital lobe	後頭葉
28	☐ parietal lobe	頭頂葉
29	☐ temporal lobe	側頭葉
30	☐ **medulla oblongata**	**延髄**

Part 3 **Terms of Body Parts and Functions** 人体各部の名称と機能の英単語

1. meninx; meningeal — 髄膜；髄膜の
2. midbrain — 中脳
3. oliva; olivary body; dentoliva — オリーブ
4. optic chiasma — 視〔神経〕交叉
5. piriform[e] sinus (fossa) — 梨状陥凹，梨状窩
6. pons — 橋
7. pyramidal decussation — 錐体交叉
8. pyramidal tract — 錐体路
9. sigmoid sinus — S状静脈洞
10. subarachnoid space — クモ膜下腔
11. subdural space — 硬膜下腔
12. sylvian fissure; lateral sulcus — シルヴィウス裂；外側溝
13. sympathetic trunk; gangliated cord — 交感神経幹
14. **thalamus**; thalamic — **視床**；視床の
15. white matter — 白質

1-6. Ear 耳

- auditory canal; external acoustic (auditory) meatus — 〔外〕耳道
- auricle; pinna — 耳介
- **cochlea** — **蝸牛**
- earlobe — 耳朶
- eustachian tube — エウスタキオ管
- external ear — 外耳
- internal ear — 内耳
- middle ear — 中耳
- otosalpinx — 耳管
- **semicircular canals** — **骨半規管**
- **tympanic membrane**; eardrum — 鼓膜

1-7. Eye 眼

- cilia; eyelashes — 睫毛(しょうもう)；まつげ
- **eye**; oculus; ocular — 目，眼；眼〔の〕
- **eyeball**; bulbus oculi — 眼球
- **eyebrow** — 眉〔毛〕
- fovea centralis — 中心窩
- **iris** — **虹彩**
- **lacrimal (lacrymal) gland** — 涙腺
- lacrimal (lacrymal) sac — 涙嚢
- **lens** — **水晶体**
- macula lutea; macula retinae; yellow spot — 黄斑
- optic disc — 視神経円板
- punctum cecum; blind spot — 盲点
- **pupil**; pupillary — **瞳孔**；瞳孔の
- **retina**; retinal — **網膜**；網膜の
- **sclera**; scleral — **強膜**；強膜の
- scotoma — 暗点
- vitreous body; hyaloid body — 硝子体

1-8. Nose 鼻

- choana — 後鼻孔
- frontal sinus — 前頭洞
- Kiesselbach area — キーセルバッハ部位(野)
- naris — 外鼻孔
- nasal cavity — 鼻腔
- nasal septum — 鼻中隔
- nasal vestibule — 鼻前庭
- **nose**; nasal — 鼻；鼻の
- nostril — 鼻孔

Part 3 **Terms of Body Parts and Functions** 人体各部の名称と機能の英単語

1. olfactory bulb — 嗅球
2. paranasal sinus — 副鼻腔
3. sphenoidal sinus — 蝶形骨洞

1-9. Mouth　口

6. frenulum linguae — 舌小帯
7. **gingiva**; gingival; **gum** — **歯肉；歯肉の；歯茎**
8. labial commissure [of mouth] — 〔口の〕唇交連
9. lingual papilla — 舌乳頭
10. **oral cavity**; **mouth** — **口腔；口**
11. **palate**; palatine — **口蓋；口蓋の**
12. hard palate — 硬口蓋
13. soft palate — 軟口蓋
14. palatine tonsil — 口蓋扁桃
15. palatine uvula — 口蓋垂
16. **salivary gland** — **唾液腺**
17. **tongue**; lingua; lingual — **舌；舌の**
18. **tooth**; dens; dental — **歯；歯の**
19. canine [tooth]; cuspid [tooth] — 犬歯
20. deciduous tooth; baby tooth — 乳歯
21. molar [tooth] — 〔大〕臼歯
22. premolar [tooth]; bicuspid [tooth] — 〔小〕臼歯
23. third molar [tooth]; wisdom tooth — 第三大臼歯；智歯；親知らず

1-10. Skin　皮膚

26. bald — 禿頭の，頭髪がない
27. beard — 顎髭
28. **cuticle** — **角質**
29. dermis; dermal — 真皮；真皮の，皮膚の
30. **epidermis**; epidermal — **表皮；表皮の**

1	☐ **foreskin**	**包皮**
2	☐ **hair**	**毛髪**
3	☐ body hair	体毛
4	☐ hair follicle	毛包
5	☐ hair root	毛根
6	☐ hair shaft	毛幹
7	☐ pubic hair	恥毛
8	☐ scalp hair	頭髪
9	☐ hairless	無毛〔性〕の
10	☐ hairy	有毛〔性〕の，毛むくじゃらの
11	☐ mustache	口髭
12	☐ **scalp**	**頭皮**
13	☐ **skin**; cutis; cutaneous	**皮膚**；皮膚の
14	☐ **sweat gland**	**汗腺**
15	☐ whiskers	頬髭

2 Back and Spinal Cord
背部と脊髄

1. ☐ **back**; dorsal — 背；背側の，背面の
2. ☐ lower back — 腰
3. ☐ **hip** — ヒップ，腰部，股関節部

2-1. Bones, Ligaments and Joints 骨・靭帯・関節

6. ☐ **intervertebral disc** — 椎間板
7. ☐ intervertebral disc space — 椎間板腔
8. ☐ intervertebral foramen — 椎間孔
9. ☐ intervertebral joint — 椎間関節
10. ☐ Luschka joint — ルシュカ関節
11. ☐ sacrum; sacral — 仙骨；仙骨の
12. ☐ **spine**; spinal — 脊椎；脊椎の，脊髄の
13. ☐ transverse process — 横突起
14. ☐ **vertebra**; vertebral — 椎骨；椎骨の
15. ☐ lumbar vertebra; lumbar spine — 腰椎
16. ☐ sacral vertebra — 仙椎
17. ☐ thoracic vertebra — 胸椎
18. ☐ vertebral arch — 椎弓
19. ☐ vertebral body — 椎体
20. ☐ vertebral canal; spinal canal — 脊柱管
21. ☐ vertebral column; dorsal spine; backbone — 脊柱；背骨
23. ☐ vertebral foramen — 椎孔
24. ☐ yellow ligament — 黄〔色〕靭帯

2-2. Muscles 筋肉

- [ ] erector spinae [muscle]　脊柱起立筋
- [ ] iliocostalis cervicis [muscle]　頚腸肋筋
- [ ] iliocostalis lumborum [muscle]　腰腸肋筋
- [ ] iliocostalis thoracis [muscle]　胸腸肋筋
- [ ] infraspinatus [muscle]　棘下筋
- [ ] latissimus dorsi [muscle]　広背筋
- [ ] multifidus [muscle]　多裂筋
- [ ] paraspinal muscle　傍脊柱筋
- [ ] psoas major [muscle]　大腰筋
- [ ] psoas minor [muscle]　小腰筋
- [ ] rhomboid major [muscle]　大菱形筋
- [ ] rhomboid minor [muscle]　小菱形筋
- [ ] rotatores [muscle]　回旋筋
- [ ] sacrospinalis [muscle]　仙棘筋
- [ ] serratus posterior inferior [muscle]　下後鋸筋
- [ ] serratus posterior superior [muscle]　上後鋸筋
- [ ] spinalis cervicis [muscle]　頚棘筋
- [ ] spinalis thoracis [muscle]　胸棘筋
- [ ] splenius capitis [muscle]　頭板状筋
- [ ] splenius cervicis [muscle]　頚板状筋
- [ ] trapezius [muscle]　僧帽筋

2-3. Nerves 神経

- [ ] anterior interosseous nerve 前骨間神経
- [ ] lumbar cord 腰髄
- [ ] lumbar nerve 腰神経
- [ ] lumbar plexus 腰神経叢
- [ ] motor nerve 運動神経
- [ ] sacral nerve 仙骨神経
- [ ] sacral plexus 仙骨神経叢
- [ ] **spinal cord** **脊髄；後根神経節**
- [ ] spinal ganglion; dorsal root ganglion 脊髄神経節
- [ ] spinal nerve 脊髄神経
- [ ] spinal segment 脊髄髄節（分節）

COLUMN 頭が痛い"頭"の英語

「頭」を表す英語はheadだけではない。またそれぞれの語が示す頭の部分が以下のように異なる。

① head（頭）：広義では首から上。狭義では，顔面を除く大脳（cerebrum, 小脳（cerebellum），脳幹（brain stem）を言う。

② caput（頭）：headと同じ。器官の頭部についてもいう（例：caput femoris 大腿骨頭）。

③ cranium, skull（頭蓋）：頭部の骨格。

④ encephalon, brain（頭髄・脳）：脳脊髄のうち，頭骸骨の中にある前脳，中脳，菱脳部分。cephalon（ギリシャ語：頭）のen（中）の意味。

⑤ cerebrum（大脳）：主として大脳半球。

それにしても，専門英語を初めて見たときは未知の外国語のようで，"It's over my head."（頭の上を飛んでいるかのように），"It's all Greek to me."（知らないギリシャ語を聞いているように）わからない，「珍粉漢粉/珍糞漢糞」（陳粉＝分，漢＝男性：中国人の名前が珍しいため）で，頭痛（headache）や片頭痛（migraine）が起きたかも知れない。また，用語の多さに頭にくる（go crazy）かも知れないが，頭を休め（rest one's mind），頭を冷やしながら（calm down）続けよう。

3 Chest
胸部

1. ☐ axillary cavity; axilla; armpit — 腋窩；腋（わき）
2. ☐ **breast** — **胸〔部〕，乳房**
3. ☐ **chest**; **thorax**; thoracic — **胸〔部〕；胸郭；胸〔郭〕の**
4. ☐ thoracic cavity — 胸腔
5. ☐ epigastrium — 心窩部，みぞおち
6. ☐ thymus [gland] — 胸腺
7. ☐ Valsalva sinus — バルサルバ洞

3-1. Bones, Ligaments and Joints 骨・靭帯・関節

10. ☐ intercostal space — 肋間隙
11. ☐ **rib**; **costa**; costal — **肋骨**；肋骨の
12. ☐ **shoulder blade**; **scapula** — **肩甲骨**
13. ☐ sternoclavicular joint — 胸鎖関節
14. ☐ sternocostal joint — 胸肋関節
15. ☐ **sternum**; sternal — **胸骨**；胸骨の
16. ☐ xiphoid process; xiphisternum — 剣状突起

3-2. Muscles 筋肉

19. ☐ **diaphragm**; diaphragmatic — **横隔膜**；横隔膜の
20. ☐ expiratory muscle — 呼息筋
21. ☐ external intercostal [muscle] — 外肋間筋
22. ☐ internal intercostal [muscle] — 内肋間筋
23. ☐ longissimus thoracis [muscle] — 胸最長筋
24. ☐ lumbar triangle; Petit triangle — 腰三角
25. ☐ pectoralis major [muscle] — 大胸筋
26. ☐ pectoralis minor [muscle] — 小胸筋
27. ☐ respiratory muscle — 呼吸筋

Part 3 **Terms of Body Parts and Functions** 人体各部の名称と機能の英単語

- [ ] serratus anterior [muscle] 前鋸筋
- [ ] sternocleidomastoid [muscle] 胸鎖乳突筋

3-3. Nerves 神経

- [ ] axillary nerve 腋窩神経
- [ ] motor root 運動神経根
- [ ] thoracic nerve 胸神経

3-4. Blood Vessels 血管

- [ ] **aorta**; aortic **大動脈**；大動脈の
- [ ]   ascending aorta 上行大動脈
- [ ]   descending aorta 下行大動脈
- [ ] aortic arch 大動脈弓
- [ ] aortic valve 大動脈弁
- [ ] **artery**; arterial **動脈**；動脈の
- [ ] brachiocephalic trunk 腕頭動脈
- [ ] **capillary** **毛細〔血〕管**
- [ ] **coronary artery** **冠状動脈**
- [ ] lymph node リンパ節
- [ ] lymph sinus リンパ洞
- [ ] lymph vessel リンパ管
- [ ] pulmonary arteries 肺動脈
- [ ] pulmonary trunk 肺動脈幹
- [ ] pulmonary valve 肺動脈弁
- [ ] right lymphatic duct 右リンパ本幹
- [ ] subclavian artery 鎖骨下動脈
- [ ] subclavian vein 鎖骨下静脈
- [ ] thoracic duct 胸管
- [ ] **vein**; venous **静脈**；静脈の

1	☐ **vena cava**	大静脈
2	☐ inferior vena cava	下大静脈
3	☐ superior vena cava	上大静脈
4	☐ venule	細静脈，小静脈
5	☐ vessel	〔脈〕管

3-5. Heart　　心臓

- ☐ apex cordis; apex of heart　　心尖
- ☐ **atrium; atrial**　　**心房；心房の**
- ☐ auricle　　心耳
- ☐ **endocardium**　　**心内膜**
- ☐ **heart; cardiac**　　**心臓；心臓の**
- ☐ **myocardium; myocardial**　　**心筋；心筋の**
- ☐ papillary muscle　　乳頭筋
- ☐ septum; septal　　中隔；中隔の
- ☐ interatrial septum　　心房中隔
- ☐ interventricular septum　　心室中隔
- ☐ tendinous cords　　腱索
- ☐ **valve**　　**弁**
- ☐ aortic valve　　大動脈弁
- ☐ mitral valve　　僧帽弁
- ☐ pulmonary valve　　肺動脈弁
- ☐ semilunar valve　　半月弁
- ☐ tricuspid valve　　三尖弁
- ☐ **ventricle; ventricular**　　**心室；心室の**
- ☐ left ventricle　　左心室
- ☐ right ventricle　　右心室

3-6. Respiratory Organs　　　呼吸器官

- ☐ alveolar sac　　肺胞囊
- ☐ **alveolus; alveolar**　　肺胞；肺胞の
- ☐ arytenoid cartilage　　披裂軟骨
- ☐ **bronchiole**; bronchiolar　　細気管支；細気管支の
- ☐ **bronchus**; bronchial　　気管支；気管支の
- ☐ cricoid cartilage　　輪状軟骨
- ☐ epiglottic cartilage　　喉頭蓋軟骨
- ☐ **epiglottis**　　喉頭蓋
- ☐ glottis　　声門
- ☐ laryngeal inlet　　喉頭口
- ☐ **larynx**; laryngeal; voice box　　喉頭；喉頭の
- ☐ **lung; pulmonary**　　肺；肺の
- ☐ **pharynx**; pharyngeal　　咽頭；咽頭の
- ☐ respiratory tract; airway　　気道
- ☐ rima glottidis　　声門裂
- ☐ rima vestibuli　　前庭裂
- ☐ **throat**　　咽喉，のど
- ☐ **trachea**; tracheal; windpipe　　気管；気管の
- ☐ tracheal bifurcation　　気管分岐部
- ☐ tracheal cartilage　　気管軟骨
- ☐ vestibular fold　　前庭ヒダ，室ヒダ
- ☐ vocal fold; vocal cord　　声帯ヒダ；声帯
- ☐ vocal ligament　　声帯靱帯

4 Abdomen and Pelvis
腹部・骨盤部

- **abdomen**; abdominal; belly; tummy 　　腹〔部〕；腹〔部〕の；お腹；ポンポン《cf. tummyは幼児語》
- flank 　　側腹〔部〕
- inguinal region; groin 　　鼡径部
- umbilicus; umbilical; belly button; navel 　　臍；臍の；へそ

4-1. Bones, Ligaments and Joints　骨・靭帯・関節

- acetabulum 　　寛骨臼
- coccygeal cornu (horn) 　　尾骨角
- coccyx; coccygeal 　　尾骨；尾骨の
- **coxal bone**; hip bone 　　**寛骨**
- **hip joint** 　　**股関節**
- ilium; iliac 　　腸骨；腸骨の
- ischium; ischial; sciatic 　　坐骨；坐骨の
- **pelvis**; pelvic 　　**骨盤**；骨盤の
- pubis; pubic 　　恥骨；恥骨の

4-2. Muscles　筋肉

- **abdominal muscle** 　　**腹筋**
- adductor brevis [muscle] 　　短内転筋
- adductor longus [muscle] 　　長内転筋
- adductor magnus [muscle] 　　大内転筋
- **anal sphincter** 　　**肛門括約筋**
- **detrusor [muscle]** 　　**排尿筋**
- external oblique [muscle] 　　外腹斜筋
- iliacus [muscle] 　　腸骨筋

- [ ] **iliopsoas [muscle]** 腸腰筋
- [ ] internal oblique [muscle] 内腹斜筋
- [ ] levator ani [muscle] 肛門挙筋
- [ ] obturator externus [muscle] 外閉鎖筋
- [ ] obturator internus [muscle] 内閉鎖筋
- [ ] pectineus [muscle] 恥骨筋
- [ ] piriformis [muscle] 梨状筋
- [ ] quadratus lumborum [muscle] 腰方形筋
- [ ] **rectus abdominis [muscle]** 腹直筋
- [ ] transversus abdominis [muscle] 腹横筋
- [ ] **urethral sphincter** 尿道括約筋
- [ ] urethrovaginal sphincter 尿道腟括約筋

4-3. Nerves 神経

- [ ] Auerbach plexus アウエルバッハ神経叢
- [ ] coccygeal nerve 尾骨神経
- [ ] pudendal nerve 陰部神経
- [ ] sciatic nerve 坐骨神経
- [ ] visceral nerve 内臓神経
- [ ] visceromotor nerve 内臓運動神経
- [ ] viscerosensory nerve 内臓感覚神経

4-4. Blood Vessels 血管

- [ ] common iliac artery 総腸骨動脈
- [ ] common iliac vein 総腸骨静脈
- [ ] renal artery 腎動脈
- [ ] splenic artery 脾動脈
- [ ] splenic vein 脾静脈
- [ ] umbilical artery 臍動脈
- [ ] umbilical vein 臍静脈

4-5. Digestive Organs　　　消化器官

- [ ] **anus**; anal　　　肛門；肛門の
- [ ] **appendix**　　　虫垂
- [ ] cardia; cardiac　　　噴門；噴門の
- [ ] cecum　　　盲腸
- [ ] **colon**　　　結腸
- [ ] common bile duct　　　総胆管
- [ ] **digestive tract; digestive tube**　　　消化管
- [ ] **duodenum**; duodenal　　　十二指腸；十二指腸の
- [ ] **esophagus**; esophageal　　　食道；食道の
- [ ] **gallbladder**; cholecyst　　　胆嚢
- [ ] ileum; ileal　　　回腸；回腸の
- [ ] **intestine**; intestinal; **bowel**; **gut**　　　腸；腸の
- [ ] 　large intestine; large bowel　　　大腸
- [ ] 　small intestine; small bowel　　　小腸
- [ ] jejunum; jejunal　　　空腸；空腸の
- [ ] **liver; hepatic**　　　肝臓；肝臓の
- [ ] muscularis　　　筋層
- [ ] **pancreas**; pancreatic　　　膵臓；膵臓の
- [ ] pancreatic duct　　　膵管
- [ ] pyloric antrum　　　幽門前庭，幽門洞
- [ ] pylorus; pyloric　　　幽門；幽門の
- [ ] **rectum**; rectal　　　直腸；直腸の
- [ ] serosa; serous　　　漿膜；漿膜の，漿液の
- [ ] **stomach; gastric**　　　胃；胃の
- [ ] submucosa　　　粘膜下層

4-6. Genitourinary Organs　　　泌尿生殖器官

- [ ] **amniotic fluid** 　羊水
- [ ] **bladder** 　膀胱
- [ ] clitoris 　陰核
- [ ] **glomerulus**; glomerular 　糸球体；糸球体の
- [ ] **kidney; renal** 　腎臓；腎臓の
- [ ] **mammary gland** 　乳腺
- [ ] **ovary**; ovarian 　卵巣；卵巣の
- [ ] **ovum**; oval 　卵子；卵子の，卵形の
- [ ] **penis**; penile 　陰茎；陰茎の
- [ ] **placenta**; placental 　胎盤；胎盤の
- [ ] **prostate gland**; prostatic 　前立腺；前立腺の
- [ ] **scrotum**; scrotal 　陰嚢；陰嚢の
- [ ] **sperm**; semen 　精子；精液
- [ ] **testis**; testicle; testicular 　精巣，睾丸；精巣の，睾丸の
- [ ] **umbilical cord** 　臍帯
- [ ] **ureter**; ureteral 　尿管；尿管の
- [ ] **urethra**; urethral 　尿道；尿道の
- [ ] uriniferous tubule; urinary tubule 　尿細管
- [ ] uterine tube; Fallopian tube 　卵管
- [ ] **uterus**; uterine; **womb** 　子宮；子宮の
- [ ] 　cervix [of uterus] 　子宮頚
- [ ] **vagina**; vaginal 　腟；腟の
- [ ] vas deferens 　〔輸〕精管

5 Upper Extremities
上肢

1. **arm** — 腕
2. upper arm; brachial; brachial — 二の腕；上腕；上腕の
3. carpus; carpal; wrist — 手根；手根の；手首
4. digit; digital; finger — 指；指の
5. **elbow** — 肘
6. eponychium — 爪上皮
7. fingerprint — 指紋
8. fist — 拳
9. **forearm** — 前腕
10. **hand; manual** — 手；手の，手動の
11. metacarpus; metacarpal — 中手；中手の
12. **nail** — 爪
13. olecranon — 肘頭
14. palm; palmar — 手掌；手掌の
15. **shoulder** — 肩
16. thenar eminence — 母指球
17. **thumb** — 母指
18. **upper extremity; upper limb** — 上肢

5-1. Bones, Ligaments and Joints
骨・靭帯・関節

21. acromion — 肩峰
22. carpometacarpal (CM) joint — 手根中手関節
23. **clavicle**; clavicular; **collar bone** — 鎖骨；鎖骨の
24. coracoid process — 烏口突起
25. **distal interphalangeal (DIP) joints** — 遠位指（趾）節間関節
26. distal radioulnar joint — 遠位（下）橈尺関節
27. **elbow joint** — 肘関節

Part 3 Terms of Body Parts and Functions 人体各部の名称と機能の英単語

1. ☐ glenohumeral joint 肩甲上腕関節
2. ☐ hamate 有鉤骨
3. ☐ hand joint 手関節
4. ☐ **humerus**; humeral **上腕骨**；上腕骨の
5. ☐ surgical neck of humerus 〔上腕骨の〕外科頸
6. ☐ intercarpal joints 手根間関節
7. ☐ Lister tubercle リスター結節
8. ☐ **metacarpal bone** **中手骨**
9. ☐ **metacarpophalangeal (MP) joints** **中手指節関節**
10. ☐ midcarpal joint 手根中央関節
11. ☐ **phalanx [of hand]** **〔手の〕指節骨**
12. ☐ pisiform 豆状骨
13. ☐ **proximal interphalangeal (PIP) joints** **近位指節間関節**
15. ☐ proximal radioulnar joint 近位(上)橈尺関節
16. ☐ radioulnar triangular cartilage 遠位橈尺関節円板
17. ☐ **radius**; radial **橈骨**；橈骨の
18. ☐ rotator cuff ローテーターカフ，
19. 〔肩〕回旋筋腱板
20. ☐ scaphoid [bone] 〔手の〕舟状骨
21. ☐ sesamoid bone [of hand] 〔手の〕種子骨
22. ☐ shoulder joint 肩関節
23. ☐ styloid process 茎状突起
24. ☐ subacromial bursa 肩峰下〔滑液〕包
25. ☐ transverse retinacular ligament 横支靭帯
26. ☐ trapezium 大菱形骨
27. ☐ trapezoid 小菱形骨
28. ☐ triquetrum 三角骨
29. ☐ **ulna**; ulnar **尺骨**；尺骨の
30. ☐ **wrist joint** **橈骨手根関節**

5-2. Muscles　　　　　　　　筋肉

- **☐ abductor [muscle]**　　**外転筋**
- ☐ abductor digiti minimi [muscle]　　小指外転筋
- ☐ abductor pollicis brevis [muscle]　　短母指外転筋
- ☐ abductor pollicis longus [muscle]　　長母指外転筋
- ☐ adductor pollicis [muscle]　　母指内転筋
- ☐ anconeus [muscle]　　肘筋
- **☐ biceps brachii [muscle]**　　**上腕二頭筋**
- **☐ brachialis [muscle]**　　**上腕筋**
- ☐ brachioradialis [muscle]　　腕橈骨筋
- ☐ coracobrachialis [muscle]　　烏口腕筋
- **☐ deltoid [muscle]**　　**三角筋**
- ☐ dorsal interossei [muscle of hand]　　〔手の〕背側骨間筋
- ☐ extensor carpi radialis brevis [muscle]　　短橈側手根伸筋
- ☐ extensor carpi radialis longus [muscle]　　長橈側手根伸筋
- ☐ extensor carpi ulnaris [muscle]　　尺側手根伸筋
- ☐ extensor digiti minimi [muscle]　　小指伸筋
- ☐ extensor digitorum muscle　　指伸筋
- ☐ extensor indicis [muscle]　　示指伸筋
- ☐ extensor pollicis brevis [muscle]　　短母指伸筋
- ☐ extensor pollicis longus [muscle]　　長母指伸筋
- ☐ flexor carpi radialis [muscle]　　橈側手根屈筋
- ☐ flexor carpi ulnaris [muscle]　　尺側手根屈筋
- ☐ flexor digiti minimi brevis [muscle]　　短小指屈筋
- ☐ flexor digitorum profundus [muscle]　　深指屈筋
- ☐ flexor digitorum superficialis [muscle]　　浅指屈筋
- ☐ flexor pollicis brevis [muscle]　　短母指屈筋

Part 3 Terms of Body Parts and Functions 人体各部の名称と機能の英単語

1. ☐ flexor pollicis longus [muscle] — 長母指屈筋
2. ☐ hypothenar muscle — 小指球筋
3. ☐ levator scapulae [muscle] — 肩甲挙筋
4. ☐ lumbricals [muscle] — 虫様筋
5. ☐ opponens digiti minimi [muscle] — 小指対立筋
6. ☐ opponens pollicis [muscle] — 母指対立筋
7. ☐ palmar interossei [muscle] — 掌側骨間筋
8. ☐ palmaris brevis [muscle] — 短掌筋
9. ☐ palmaris longus [muscle] — 長掌筋
10. ☐ pronator quadratus [muscle] — 方形回内筋
11. ☐ pronator teres [muscle] — 円回内筋
12. ☐ subclavius [muscle] — 鎖骨下筋
13. ☐ subscapularis [muscle] — 肩甲下筋
14. ☐ supinator [muscle] — 回外筋
15. ☐ supraspinatus [muscle] — 棘上筋
16. ☐ teres major [muscle] — 大円筋
17. ☐ teres minor [muscle] — 小円筋
18. ☐ thenar muscle — 母指球筋
19. ☐ **triceps branchii [muscle]** — **上腕三頭筋**

5-3. Nerves 神経

22. ☐ axillary nerve — 腋窩神経
23. ☐ brachial plexus — 腕神経叢
24. ☐ **carpal tunnel** — **手根管**
25. ☐ Guyon canal — ギヨン管
26. ☐ **median nerve** — **正中神経**
27. ☐ posterior interosseous nerve — 後骨間神経
28. ☐ **radial nerve** — **橈骨神経**
29. ☐ **ulnar nerve** — **尺骨神経**

5-4. Blood Vessels 血管

- [ ] brachial artery　　　　　上腕動脈
- [ ] brachial vein　　　　　　上腕静脈
- [ ] deep digital veins　　　　指の深静脈
- [ ] deep palmar arch　　　　深掌動脈弓
- [ ] palmar digital arteries　　掌側指動脈
- [ ] radial artery　　　　　　橈骨動脈
- [ ] radial vein　　　　　　　橈骨静脈
- [ ] superficial palmar arch　　浅掌動脈弓
- [ ] ulnar artery　　　　　　尺骨動脈
- [ ] ulnar vein　　　　　　　尺骨静脈

6 Lower Extremities
下肢

1. **buttocks**; bottom; arse; ass — 殿部《*cf.* arse, assは俗語》
2. **calf** — 腓腹，ふくらはぎ
3. **calx**; heel — 踵（かかと）
4. **femur**; femoral; thigh — 大腿；大腿の
5. **foot**; pes — 足
6. great toe — 母趾
7. hind foot — 後足部
8. **instep** — 足の甲
9. **knee**; genu — 膝
10. **leg** — 脚（あし）
11. **lower extremity**; lower limb — 下肢
12. **malleolus**; malleolar — 果（踝），くるぶし；踝の，くるぶしの
14. lateral malleolus — 外果，そとくるぶし
15. medial malleolus — 内果，うちくるぶし
16. **metatarsus**; metatarsal — 中足；中足の
17. popliteal fossa — 膝窩
18. **shin** — 脛（すね）
19. sole; plantar — 足底，足の裏；足底の
20. **tarsus**; tarsal; ankle — 足根；足根の；足首
21. **toe** — 足ゆび（指，趾）

6-1. Bones, Ligaments and Joints 骨・靭帯・関節

24. arch of foot — 足アーチ
25. ball and socket ankle joint — 球状足関節
26. **calcaneal tendon**; Achilles tendon — 踵骨腱；アキレス腱
27. **calcaneus**; calcaneal — 踵骨；踵骨の

1	☐ collateral ligament	側副靭帯
2	☐ **cruciate ligament**	**十字靭帯**
3	☐ anterior cruciate ligament	前十字靭帯
4	☐ posterior cruciate ligament	後十字靭帯
5	☐ cuboid	立方骨
6	☐ femoral neck	大腿骨頚部
7	☐ femorotibial angle	大腿脛骨角
8	☐ **femur**; **thigh bone**	**大腿骨**
9	☐ **fibula**; fibular	**腓骨**；腓骨の
10	☐ greater trochanter	大転子
11	☐ greater tubercle (tuberosity)	大結節
12	☐ iliotibial tract	腸脛靭帯
13	☐ intertarsal joints	足根間関節
14	☐ knee joint	膝関節
15	☐ lesser trochanter	小転子
16	☐ longitudinal ligaments	縦靭帯
17	☐ anterior longitudinal ligament	前縦靭帯
18	☐ posterior longitudinal ligament	後縦靭帯
19	☐ **meniscus**	**半月板，メニスクス**
20	☐ metatarsal arch	中足アーチ
21	☐ **metatarsal bone**	**中足骨**
22	☐ **metatarso-phalangeal (MTP) joints**	**中足趾節関節**
23	☐ **navicular**	〔足の〕舟状骨
24	☐ **patella**; patellar; **kneecap**	**膝蓋骨**：膝蓋骨の：膝がしら
25	☐ patellar tendon	膝蓋腱
26	☐ patellofemoral (PF) joint	膝蓋大腿関節
27	☐ pelvic girdle; hip girdle	下肢帯
28	☐ phalanx [of foot]	〔足の〕趾節骨
29	☐ posterior meniscofemoral ligament; Wrisberg ligament	後半月大腿靭帯；ヴリスベルク靭帯

Part 3 **Terms of Body Parts and Functions**　人体各部の名称と機能の英単語

1. ☐ sesamoid bone [of foot]　〔足の〕種子骨
2. ☐ subtalar joint　距骨下関節
3. ☐ talar tilt　距骨傾斜
4. ☐ talocalcaneonavicular joint　距踵舟関節
5. ☐ talocrural joint　距腿関節
6. ☐ **talus**; talar; **ankle bone**　**距骨**；距骨の
7. ☐ tarsal [bones]　足根骨
8. ☐ tarsometatarsal joints; Lisfranc joints　足根中足関節；リスフラン関節
10. ☐ **tibia**; tibial　**脛骨**；脛骨の
11. ☐ transverse tarsal joint; Chopart joint　横足根関節；ショパール関節

6-2. Muscles　筋肉

- ☐ abductor digiti minimi [muscle]　小趾外転筋
- ☐ abductor hallucis [muscle]　母趾外転筋
- ☐ adductor [muscle]　内転筋
- ☐ adductor hallucis [muscle]　母趾内転筋
- ☐ adductor tubercle　内転筋結節
- ☐ biceps femoris [muscle]; biceps muscle of thigh　大腿二頭筋
- ☐ calf muscles　腓腹筋群
- ☐ dorsal interossei [muscle of foot]　〔足の〕背側骨間筋
- ☐ extensor digitorum brevis [muscle]　短趾伸筋
- ☐ extensor digitorum longus [muscle]　長趾伸筋
- ☐ extensor hallucis brevis [muscle]　短母趾伸筋
- ☐ extensor hallucis longus [muscle]　長母趾伸筋
- ☐ fibularis brevis [muscle]　短腓骨筋
- ☐ fibularis longus [muscle]　長腓骨筋
- ☐ fibularis tertius [muscle]　第3腓骨筋

1	☐ flexor digiti minimi brevis [muscle]	短小趾屈筋
2	☐ flexor digitorum brevis [muscle]	短趾屈筋
3	☐ flexor digitorum longus [muscle]	長趾屈筋
4	☐ flexor hallucis brevis [muscle]	短母趾屈筋
5	☐ flexor hallucis longus [muscle]	長母趾屈筋
6	☐ gastrocnemius [muscle]	腓腹筋
7	☐ gluteus maximus [muscle]	大殿筋
8	☐ gluteus medius [muscle]	中殿筋
9	☐ gluteus minimus [muscle]	小殿筋
10	☐ gracilis [muscle]	薄筋
11	☐ **hamstring [muscles]**	**ハムストリング，膝屈筋〔群〕**
12	☐ inferior gemellus [muscle]	下双子筋
13	☐ opponens digiti minimi	小趾対立筋
14	pedis [muscle]	
15	☐ plantar fascia	足底腱膜
16	☐ plantar interossei [muscle]	底側骨間筋
17	☐ plantaris [muscle]	足底筋
18	☐ popliteus [muscle]	膝窩筋
19	☐ quadratus femoris [muscle]	大腿方形筋
20	☐ quadriceps femoris [muscle]	大腿四頭筋
21	☐ rectus femoris [muscle]	大腿直筋
22	☐ soleus [muscle]	ヒラメ筋
23	☐ superior gemellus [muscle]	上双子筋
24	☐ tensor fasciae latae [muscle]	大腿筋膜張筋
25	☐ tibialis anterior [muscle]	前脛骨筋
26	☐ tibialis posterior [muscle]	後脛骨筋
27	☐ triceps [muscle] of calf	下腿三頭筋
28	☐ vastus intermedius [muscle]	中間広筋
29	☐ vastus lateralis [muscle]	外側広筋
30	☐ vastus medialis [muscle]	内側広筋

Part 3 **Terms of Body Parts and Functions** 人体各部の名称と機能の英単語

6-3. Nerves 神経

- [ ] common peroneal (fibular) nerve 総腓骨神経
- [ ] deep peroneal (fibular) nerve 深腓骨神経
- [ ] femoral nerve 大腿神経
- [ ] lateral femoral cutaneous nerve 外側大腿皮神経
- [ ] obturator nerve 閉鎖神経
- [ ] saphenous nerve 伏在神経
- [ ] superficial peroneal (fibular) nerve 浅腓骨神経
- [ ] superior gluteal nerve 上殿神経
- [ ] sural nerve 腓腹神経
- [ ] tibial nerve 脛骨神経

6-4. Blood Vessels 血管

- [ ] dorsalis pedis artery 足背動脈
- [ ] femoral artery 大腿動脈
- [ ] femoral vein 大腿静脈
- [ ] popliteal artery 膝窩動脈
- [ ] popliteal lymph nodes 膝窩リンパ節
- [ ] popliteal vein 膝窩静脈
- [ ] saphenous vein 伏在静脈

7 Histology
組織学用語

7-1. Blood Cells 血液細胞

- [ ] **erythrocyte**; red blood cell (RBC) — 赤血球
- [ ] **leukocyte**; white blood cell (WBC) — 白血球
- [ ] **lymphocyte** — リンパ球
- [ ] **macrophage** — 貪食細胞，マクロファージ
- [ ] **plasma** — 血漿
- [ ] **platelet** — 血小板
- [ ] **serum** — 血清
- [ ] **spleen**; splenic — 脾臓；脾臓の
  - [ ] red pulp of spleen — 赤脾髄
  - [ ] white pulp of spleen — 白脾髄

7-2. Tumors 腫瘍

- [ ] **cancer** — がん，癌腫
- [ ] carcinoid — カルチノイド，類癌腫
- [ ] **carcinoma** — 癌腫
  - [ ] basal cell carcinoma — 基底細胞がん
  - [ ] squamous cell carcinoma — 扁平上皮がん
- [ ] **growth** — 増殖，腫瘍
- [ ] hyperplasia — 過形成
- [ ] lymphoma — リンパ腫
- [ ] **neoplasm** — 新生物
- [ ] pseudolymphoma — 偽リンパ腫
- [ ] **sarcoma** — 肉腫
- [ ] **tumor** — 腫瘍，腫瘤，腫脹

Part 3 **Terms of Body Parts and Functions**　人体各部の名称と機能の英単語

8　Physiology
生理学用語

8-1. Head and Neck　頭頚部

- audition; hearing　聴覚
- auditory (hearing) acuity　聴力
- auditory sensation area　可聴範囲
- auditory threshold　可聴閾値
- cerebral circulation　脳循環
- cerebral perfusion pressure　脳灌流圧
- cerebral plasticity　脳の可塑性
- **cerebrospinal fluid (CSF)**　**〔脳脊〕髄液**
- color sensation　色覚
- conjugate gaze　共同〔性〕注視
- conjugate movement of eyes　眼球共同運動
- dark adaptation　暗順応
- **field of vision**　**視野**
- gaze　注視
- light sensation　光覚
- local cerebral blood volume　局所脳血液量
- local cerebral glucose utilization　局所脳ブドウ糖消費
- local cerebral metabolic rate of glucose　局所脳ブドウ糖代謝率
- local cerebral metabolic rate of oxygen　局所脳酸素消費量
- miosis　縮瞳
- ocular movement　眼球運動
- orthophoria　眼球正位
- perception of three dimensional space　三次元空間知覚

1	☐ **sleep**	睡眠
2	☐ non-rapid eye movement (NREM) sleep	ノンREM睡眠
3	☐ rapid eye movement (REM) sleep	レム睡眠
4	☐ sleep architecture	睡眠構造
5	☐ sleep cycle	睡眠周期
6	☐ sleep efficiency	睡眠効率
7	☐ sleep onset	睡眠開始
8	☐ sleep onset REM period	睡眠開始(入眠)時レム期
9	☐ sleep stage	睡眠段階
10	☐ spatial visual acuity	空間視力
11	☐ **swallowing; deglutition**	**嚥下**
12	☐ swallowing function	嚥下機能
13	☐ taste	味覚
14	☐ vestibular sense	前庭感覚
15	☐ **visual acuity**	**視力**
16	☐ visual angle	視角
17	☐ visual feedback	視覚フィードバック
18	☐ visual sense (sensation)	視覚

8-2. Back and Spinal Cord　　背部と脊髄

21	☐ intradiscal pressure	椎間板内圧
22	☐ spinal motor neuron	脊髄運動ニューロン

8-3. Chest　　胸部

25	☐ alveolar ventilation	肺胞換気
26	☐ dead space	死腔
27	☐ functional dead space	生理的死腔
28	☐ **expiration**	**呼息**
29	☐ **gas exchange**	**ガス交換**
30	☐ **inspiration**	**吸息**

Part 3 **Terms of Body Parts and Functions** 人体各部の名称と機能の英単語

☐ **oxygen consumption**	**酸素消費〔量〕**
☐ myocardial oxygen consumption	心筋酸素消費量
☐ oxygen dissociation curve	酸素解離曲線
☐ oxygen uptake (intake)	酸素摂取〔量〕
☐ myocardial oxygen uptake	心筋酸素摂取量
☐ pulmonary function	肺機能
☐ **respiration; respiratory**	**呼吸;呼吸の**
☐ abdominal respiration	腹式呼吸
☐ spontaneuos respiration	自発呼吸
☐ thoracic respiration	胸式呼吸
☐ respiratory function	呼吸機能
☐ respiratory quotient	呼吸商
☐ respiratory sound	呼吸音
☐ saturation of hemoglobin with oxygen (SaO$_2$)	酸素飽和度

8-4. Abdomen and Pelvis 腹部・骨盤部

☐ abdominal pressure	腹圧
☐ **defecation**	**排便**
☐ hepatic blood flow	肝血流量
☐ **urination; voiding; micturition**	**排尿**
☐ micturition desire	尿意
☐ voluntary micturition	随意排尿
☐ **urine; uric; urinary**	**尿;尿の**
☐ residual urine	残尿

8-5. Upper Extremities 上肢

☐ ambidexterity	両手利き
☐ left handed; sinistromanual	左手利きの
☐ right handed; dextromanual	右手利きの

8-6. Reactions, Reflexes and Responses 反応，反射

- [ ] **reaction** 反応
- [ ]   alerting reaction 警告反応
- [ ]   indirect pupillary reaction 間接瞳孔反応
- [ ]   near reaction 近見反応
- [ ]   Peiper-Isbert reaction パイパーーイスバート反応
- [ ]   placing reaction 踏み直り反応
- [ ]   postural reaction 姿勢反応
- [ ] **reflex** 反射
- [ ]   abdominal reflex 腹壁反射
- [ ]   Achilles tendon reflex (ATR); triceps surae reflex アキレス腱反射；下腿三頭筋反射
- [ ]   anal reflex 肛門反射
- [ ]   aponeurotic reflex 足底腱膜反射
- [ ]   asymmetric tonic neck reflex (ATNR) 非対称性緊張性頚反射
- [ ]   Babinski reflex バビンスキー反射
- [ ]   biceps femoris reflex 大腿二頭筋反射
- [ ]   biceps reflex 二頭筋反射
- [ ]   blink reflex 瞬目反射
- [ ]   calcaneal reflex 踵骨反射
- [ ]   chin (jaw) reflex 下顎反射
- [ ]   conjunctival reflex 結膜反射
- [ ]   corneal reflex 角膜反射
- [ ]   cough reflex 咳嗽反射
- [ ]   cremasteric reflex 挙睾筋反射
- [ ]   deltoid reflex 三角筋反射
- [ ]   external oblique reflex 外腹斜筋反射
- [ ]   facial reflex 顔面筋反射
- [ ]   faucial reflex 口峡反射
- [ ]   flexion reflex 屈曲反射

Part 3 **Terms of Body Parts and Functions** 人体各部の名称と機能の英単語

1	flexor reflex	屈筋反射
2	gag reflex	嘔吐反射，催吐反射
3	Gonda reflex	ゴンダ反射
4	grasp[ing] reflex	把握反射，握り反射
5	head retraction reflex	頭後屈反射
6	Hoffmann reflex	ホフマン反射
7	laryngeal reflex	喉頭反射
8	light reflex	対光反射
9	masseter reflex	咬筋反射
10	Mendel-Bechterew reflex	メンデル-ベヒテレフ反射
11	micturition reflex	排尿反射
12	near reflex	近見反射
13	Oppenheim reflex	オッペンハイム反射
14	optical winking reflex; wink reflex	〔視性〕瞬目反射
15	orbicularis oculi reflex	眼輪筋反射
16	palatal (palatine) reflex	〔軟〕口蓋反射
17	patellar tendon reflex (PTR)	膝蓋腱反射
18	pathologic reflex	病的反射
19	pharyngeal reflex	咽頭反射
20	plantar muscle reflex	足底筋反射
21	plantar reflex	足底反射
22	postural reflex	姿勢反射
23	pupillary reflex	瞳孔反射
24	rectal reflex	直腸反射
25	Rossolimo reflex	ローソリモ反射
26	Schaeffer reflex	シェファー反射
27	skin reflex	皮膚反射
28	snout reflex	口尖らし反射
29	spinal reflex	脊髄反射
30	spinobulbospinal reflex	脊髄延髄脊髄反射

1	☐ stepping reflex	足踏み反射
2	☐ stretch reflex	伸長反射
3	☐ suprapubic extensor reflex	恥骨上伸展反射
4	☐ swallowing reflex	嚥下反射
5	☐ symmetrical tonic neck reflex	対称性緊張性頚反射
6	☐ tendon reflex	腱反射
7	☐ toe reflex	足趾反射
8	☐ triceps reflex; elbow reflex	上腕三頭筋反射；肘反射
9	☐ Trömner reflex	トレムナー反射
10	☐ vestibular postural reflex	前庭姿勢反射
11	☐ vestibular reflex	前庭反射
12	☐ vestibulospinal reflex	前庭脊髄反射
13	☐ vomiting reflex; retching reflex	嘔吐反射
14	☐ **response**	**反応，応答**
15	☐ arousal response (reaction)	覚醒応答(反応)
16	☐ best motor response (BMR)	最良運動反応
17	☐ hopping response	跳び直り反応
18	☐ startle response	驚愕反応
19	☐ stepping response	足踏み反応

8-7. Physiologically Active Substances　生体分子，生理活性物質

22	☐ **adrenaline; epinephrine**	アドレナリン；エピネフリン
23	☐ **amino acid**	アミノ酸
24	☐ **antibody**	抗体
25	☐ **antigen**	抗原
26	☐ **cholesterol**	コレステロール
27	☐ **enzyme**	酵素
28	☐ **fatty acid**	脂肪酸
29	☐ **folic acid**	葉酸
30	☐ **glucose**	ブドウ糖

Part 3 Terms of Body Parts and Functions　人体各部の名称と機能の英単語

- **hormone** — ホルモン
  - adrenocorticotropic hormone (ACTH) — 副腎皮質刺激ホルモン
  - antidiuretic hormone (ADH); vasopressin — 抗利尿ホルモン；バソプレシン
  - gonadotropic hormone; gonadotropin — 性腺刺激ホルモン
  - gonadotropin-releasing hormone (GRH, GnRH) — 性腺刺激ホルモン放出ホルモン
  - growth hormone (GH) — 成長ホルモン
  - luteinizing hormone (LH) — 黄体形成（黄体化）ホルモン
  - parathyroid hormone (PTH) — 副甲状腺ホルモン
  - thyroid-stimulating hormone (TSH); thyrotropin — 甲状腺刺激ホルモン
  - thyrotropin-releasing hormone (TRH) — 甲状腺刺激ホルモン放出ホルモン
- **immunoglobulin (Ig)** — 免疫グロブリン
- **insulin** — インスリン
- **lactose** — 乳糖
  - niacin — ナイアシン
  - noradrenaline; norepinephrine — ノルアドレナリン；ノルエピネフリン
- **polysaccharide** — 多糖類
- **protein** — たんぱく（蛋白）〔質〕
- **uric acid** — 尿酸
- **vitamin** — ビタミン

COLUMN　名詞とは似ても似つかない形容詞

器官名の形容詞には，元の名詞からは想像もつかないものがある。その一例を挙げよう。

	英語名詞	形容詞	専門用語(特に記載がないものはラテン語)
1. 口	mouth	oral	os
2. 耳	ear	aural	auris
3. 手	hand	manual	manus (manualis)
4. 足	foot	pedal	pes
5. 歯	tooth	dental	dens
6. 胃	stomach	gastric	gaster (ギリシャ語)
7. 肝臓	liver	hepatic	hepar (ギリシャ語)
8. 心臓	heart	cardiac	cardia (ギリシャ語)
9. 脳	brain	cerebra	cerebrum
10.肺	lung	pulmonary	pulmo

もちろん英語はstomach ulcer(胃潰瘍)のように名詞を並べ複合語を形成する。けれども，gastric ulcerとも言うし，胃洗浄はgastric lavage (irrigation)としか言わない。多くの医学英語が，上記右欄のギリシャ語やラテン語に由来する語を借用していることから，形容詞もまた，それに準じて作られたと考えられる。

いずれにせよ，形容詞は表現を限定もするし，また豊かにする働きをもつ。医療の英語にあるさまざまな形容詞に気をつけてみるのも面白いであろう。

Part 4

Useful Expressions for Rehabilitation

リハビリテーションに役立つ
英語表現

1 Activities of Daily Living (ADL)
日常生活動作

1-1. Interview　面接

- [ ] chief complaint (CC)　主訴
- [ ] family history (FH)　家族歴
- [ ] history of present illness (PI, HPI)　現病歴
- [ ] marital history (MH)　結婚歴
- [ ] past history (PH)　既往歴
- [ ] social history (SH)　社会歴
- [ ] systemic review (SR)　病歴要約，系統別調査
- [ ] allergic history (AH)　アレルギー歴
- [ ] drug history (DH)　薬歴

A. First time interview / First session　初回面接

- [ ] ① I am Morita, your physical therapist.
  担当になりました理学療法士の森田と申します。
- [ ] ② I take care of you in walking, reducing the pain, recovering your body function in movement.
  私は歩いたり，痛みを和らげたり，運動機能の回復を担当します。
- [ ] ③ Let's start rehabilitation together.
  これから一緒にリハビリを進めていきましょう。
- [ ] ④ As this is the first time, may I ask you some questions?
  初めてなので，いくつかお聞かせ願えますか？
- [ ] ⑤ What is the most in need for you at present?
  今一番困っていることは何ですか？

Part 4 **Useful Expressions for Rehabilitation**　リハビリテーションに役立つ英語表現

- ⑥ Where is the most painful part?
  一番痛いところはどこですか？《整形外科疾患の場合》
- ⑦ When did the condition start?
  その状態はいつから始まりましたか？
- ⑧ How and where does it hurt?
  どこがどんなふうに痛みますか？
- ⑨ How was the situation of your numbness?
  How severe was your numbness?
  麻痺はどんな状態でしたか？
- ⑩ Did you have any disease before?
  他に過去にかかった病気はありますか？
- ⑪ Let me ask you about your family.
  ご家族のことについてお尋ねします。
- ⑫ Who do you live with?
  どなたと一緒に住んでいますか？
- ⑬ Who looks after you most?
  Who do you rely on most?
  どなたが一番力に（親身に）なってくれますか？
- ⑭ What do you do? / What is your job?
  ご職業は何ですか？
- ⑮ What are your hobbies?
  趣味は何ですか？
- ⑯ How do you spend a day?
  一日をどのように過ごしておられますか？

B. Afterward second session　2回目以降

- ① Good morning.
  おはようございます。
- ② Good afternoon.
  こんにちは。

- ③ How is it going?
  How is everything going?
  Is everything all right?
  調子はどうですか？（お加減はいかがですか？）
- ④ Is there anything different from last time?
  何か変わったことはありますか？
- ⑤ Now we are going to do MMT (manual muscle test) to measure the power of muscle.
  筋力を測るためにMMT（徒手筋力テスト）をします。
- ⑥ Please lie down on your back on this bed.
  では，こちらのベッドにあおむけに寝てください。
- ⑦ Let's do sit-up exercise three times.
  起き上がり運動を3回やりましょう。
- ⑧ Do bending and stretching exercise five times.
  屈曲伸展運動を5回してください。
- ⑨ Now I am going to measure the bending power of your body muscles.
  これから，身体を曲げる力を測ります。
- ⑩ Please raise your upper-body with stretching your hands when I give a sign.
  合図をしたら，手を前に伸ばしながら身体を持ち上げてください。
- ⑪ Clasp your hands behind your head.
  手を頭の後ろで組んでください。
- ⑫ Now I will measure your muscular strength to raise your legs outward.
  これから脚を外側に上げる力を測ります。
- ⑬ Please keep stopping your leg at this position as I will put resistance to it.
  抵抗を加えますので，脚をこの位置で止めていてください。

Part 4 **Useful Expressions for Rehabilitation**　リハビリテーションに役立つ英語表現

1-2. Transfer Activities　移乗・移動動作

- [ ] lie down　横になる
- [ ] lay down　横にさせる
- [ ] get up　起きる
- [ ] set up　起こす
- [ ] move along　動かす
- [ ] insert the sliding (transfer) board under ...
   …の下にスライディングボードを入れる
- [ ] pull out the sliding (transfer) board
   スライディングボードを引っぱる
- [ ] push a wheelchair　車椅子を押す
- [ ] transfer *sb* out of ...
   人を…から移乗させる（*sb* = somebody）
- [ ] transfer *sb* into (onto) ...　人を…へ移乗させる
- [ ] turn over　寝返る
- [ ] lean forward　前かがみになる
- [ ] sit back in a wheelchair　車椅子に深く座る
- [ ] sit up straight　まっすぐ座る

- [ ] ① Could you get up (lie down) on the bed?
   ベッドから起きて（横になって）いただけますか。
- [ ] ② The height of the bed is adjusted to the same level of your chair just beside it.
   ベッドの高さは傍の椅子の高さに合わせています。
- [ ] ③ Bend the knee of the opposite side, you will get up, turn over and then, sit up supporting your body with your leg.
   起き上がる方向と反対の膝を立てて、寝がえりを打ち、足の力を使いながら、起き上がってください。

- ④ Let me spread a sliding seat on the bed and roll over your body to me.
  ベッドの上にスライディングシートを広げますので，私の方へ身体を回転させてください。
- ⑤ Let me insert the sliding [transfer] board under your buttocks.
  お尻の下にスライディングボードを入れさせてください。
- ⑥ Please lean your upper part of your body to one side and forward at the same time.
  上半身を横に傾け，同時に前かがみになってください。
- ⑦ The arm support of the wheelchair is already taken away for you to slide yourself on the board to the seat.
  車椅子のアームサポートはもう外されていますから，ボードからシートに身体を滑らせてください。
- ⑧ Sit back in the seat not to fall out of the chair.
  席に深く座り落ちないようにしてください。
- ⑨ Pull out the transfer board for yourself, if you can.
  もしできれば，自分でスライディングボードを引っ張ってください。
- ⑩ We prepare some transferring devices such as hoist, stair-lift or sling for a person who can't walk.
  歩けない人のために，移動のための装置，例えば，ホイスト，階段昇降機，スリングを用意しています。
- ⑪ We can help you move from the bed to a wheelchair by using a hoist.
  ホイストを使って，ベッドから車椅子へ移動するお手伝いをします。
- ⑫ Could you move your wheelchair along the bed?
  車椅子をベッドづたいに動かしていただけますか。
- ⑬ Will you walk around with a cane?
  杖をついて歩きましょうか。
- ⑭ You are lopsided in the chair so I'll help you sit straight.
  椅子からずり落ちていますから，まっすぐに座るようにします。

Part 4 **Useful Expressions for Rehabilitation** リハビリテーションに役立つ英語表現

☐ ⑮ Shall (May) I push your wheelchair to the dining room?
食堂まで車椅子を押していきましょうか。

1-3. Housework Activities　家事動作
A. Cleaning　掃除

- ☐ do household (domestic) chores; keep house　家事をする
- ☐ defend mishaps (potential dangers)
  不運な事故（潜在的な事故）を防止する
- ☐ make the breakfast　朝食をつくる
- ☐ wash rice　米を研ぐ
- ☐ pare a potato　ジャガイモの皮をむく
- ☐ peel an orange　みかんの皮をむく
- ☐ chop up　刻む
- ☐ put some water in ...　〜に水を入れる
- ☐ take out the garbage　ごみを出す
- ☐ clean the house　家の掃除をする
- ☐ sweep the floor　床をはく
- ☐ wing out a damp cloth　（ねじって）雑巾をしぼる
- ☐ mop the floor　床にモップをかける
- ☐ do the laundry　洗濯をする
- ☐ dry clothes in the sun　洗濯物を外に干す
- ☐ dry clothes in the dryer　洗濯物を乾燥機で乾かす
- ☐ hang (peg) laundry (the washing out)
  洗濯物を干す（洗濯バサミでとめる）
- ☐ smooth the wrinkles　しわをのばす
- ☐ fold the laundry　洗濯物をたたむ

- ☐ ① Pull the handle of the window sash and let some fresh air in.
  サッシ用取っ手を引っ張って窓を開け，きれいな空気を入れましょう。
- ☐ ② Folding dust cloth and wiping the floor with all your strength is effective exercises for your stiff fingers.
  雑巾をたたんで力いっぱい床を拭くことは，硬くなった指の運動に効果的です。
- ☐ ③ Mopping the floor is easier than sweeping it with a broom or by a heavy vacuum cleaner.
  床をモップで拭く方が，ほうきで床をはいたり，重い掃除機をかけたりするよりも簡単です。
- ☐ ④ Please put your one hand on the edge of the bathtub whenever you wash the inside with a sponge.
  浴槽の内側を洗うときは，必ず片手で浴槽の縁につかまってください。
- ☐ ⑤ Don't work too hard at cleaning every day.
  毎日の掃除であまり無理をしないでください。

B. Cooking　調理

- ☐ ① Lean over the [kitchen] counter to support yourself.
  身体を支えるために台所のカウンターに寄りかかってください。
- ☐ ② You can cut vegetables with the knife with a grip and non-slip chopping board easier and in safe.
  グリップつきの包丁と滑らないまな板で，より容易に安全に野菜を切ることができます。
- ☐ ③ Press the button of the microwave oven with your unaffected hand.
  電子レンジのボタンを患部でない方の手で押してください。
- ☐ ④ Let's go to the supermarket nearby here to buy insufficient foods.
  近くのスーパーマーケットへ足りない食物を買いに行きましょう。

Part 4 **Useful Expressions for Rehabilitation**　リハビリテーションに役立つ英語表現

C. Washing clothes　洗濯

- ① Let us help you do the laundry, dry in the sun, and take it in.
  洗濯をして，外に干し，取り入れるお手伝いをします．
- ② Lean against the washing machine when you put your laundry in and out.
  洗濯物の出し入れのときは，洗濯機にもたれてください．
- ③ Pick up (Catch up) the laundry from the washer by [handling] the reacher.
  リーチャーを使って洗濯機から洗濯物を出してください．
- ④ As it is bad weather today, you should dry the laundry in the washing drier.
  今日は天気が悪いので，洗濯物は乾燥機で乾かした方がいいです．
- ⑤ For the time being, ironing the clothes is dangerous for you.
  今のところ，アイロンがけをするのは危険です．

D. Shopping　買物

- ① A care worker will visit you around at one [o'clock] in the afternoon.
  ケアワーカーが午後1時ごろ訪問します．
- ② She will bring you to the supermarket by her car.
  彼女が車でスーパーマーケットへ連れて行ってくれます．
- ③ Don't worry. She will help you shop some foods and goods.
  心配いりません．彼女が食べ物や品物を買うのを手伝います．
- ④ Please take notes of goods you want to buy there.
  どうぞそこで買う物をメモしてください．
- ⑤ Shopping will be a start for you to live independently at home.
  買物することで，あなたが家で自立した生活を始めることになります．

E. Other activities　その他

- ① There are many potential dangers in doing household chores.
  家事をするとき，多くの危険が隠れています。
- ② Preventing accidents is the first thing you should pay attention to.
  事故防止をまず注意しなければなりません。
- ③ Every housework activity is a good physical training for you.
  あらゆる家事が，あなたには良い身体運動トレーニングです。
- ④ Many convenient self-help devices will help your activities at home.
  多くの便利な自助具が自宅での活動の助けになります。
- ⑤ For example, a reacher can be used in such activities as putting your clothes on and off, catching things on the floor or pressing switches.
  例えば，リーチャーは，洋服の着脱，床の物を取ったり，スイッチを押したり，というような動作に使われます。

1-4. Dressing Activities　更衣動作

- put on one's gown　ガウンをはおる
- put on socks　靴下を穿く
- put on (off) ...　～を着る（脱ぐ）《動作》
- take on (off) ...　～を身に着ける（外す）《動作》
- wear; have on　服などを身につけている《状態》
- put on (take off) one's hat　帽子をかぶる（脱ぐ）
- put on (take off) one's glasses　メガネをかける（外す）
- put in (insert) one's contact lenses
  コンタクトレンズをはめる
- put (take) out one's contact lenses
  コンタクトレンズを外す

Part 4 **Useful Expressions for Rehabilitation** リハビリテーションに役立つ英語表現

- [ ] change one's clothes; change into ... 〔…に〕着替える
- [ ] dress in 正装している《状態》
- [ ] tie up; fasten / loosen 締める / 緩める
- [ ] button / unbutton ボタンをはめる / ボタンを外す
- [ ] zip up / unzip ジッパーを閉める / 開ける

- [ ] ① May I help you take off your clothes?
  服を脱ぐのをお手伝いしましょうか？
- [ ] ② Let's put on your pajamas.
  パジャマを着ましょう。
- [ ] ③ This button aid is helpful to button your pajama top.
  このボタンエイドはパジャマの上着のボタンをかけるのに役立ちます。
- [ ] ④ You don't have to put on in a mad rush, we've got time.
  慌てて着なくてもいいですよ。急いでいるわけじゃないですから。
- [ ] ⑤ Let's put on the pajama bottoms.
  パジャマのズボンを穿きましょう。
- [ ] ⑥ Sit down on the edge of the bed.
  ベッドの端に座ってください。
- [ ] ⑦ Cross your affected leg on the other.
  患足をもう一方の足の上に組んでください。
- [ ] ⑧ Place your hands on my shoulders and lift your right leg.
  私の肩に両手を置いて，右脚を上げてください。
- [ ] ⑨ Please put your foot into one of the pajamas halfway.
  片脚を途中まで入れてください。
- [ ] ⑩ Hold the upper part of the bottoms, and pull it up.
  ズボンの上部分を持って立ち，そこを引っ張ってください。
- [ ] ⑪ That's it. Great! You did it.
  そうです。うまい！ できました。

- ☐ ⑫ You are easily able to put on socks with this aid.
  この補助具を使ってソックスを簡単に穿けます。
- ☐ ⑬ Pull up the strings attached to the sock aid.
  ソックス補助具についている紐を引っ張ってください。
- ☐ ⑭ Are you itchy anywhere?
  どこか痒いところはないですか。
- ☐ ⑮ If possible, fold up your clothes.
  できれば、服をたたんでください。

1-5. Feeding Activities　食事動作

- ☐ eat; have; take　食べる
- ☐ gobble up　急いで食べる，丸呑みする
- ☐ drink　飲む
- ☐ chew; masticate　咀嚼する
- ☐ swallow　嚥下する
- ☐ choke　むせる
- ☐ get stuck　詰まる
- ☐ quench　潤す
- ☐ cut　切る
- ☐ mix　混ぜる
- ☐ tear　裂く
- ☐ dip　浸す
- ☐ serve the food; meal　配膳する

- ☐ ① It's time for breakfast.
  朝ごはんの時間です。
- ☐ ② Please sit down at the table.
  どうぞ、食卓についてください。
- ☐ ③ Let me set the lapboard on your bed.

Part 4 **Useful Expressions for Rehabilitation** リハビリテーションに役立つ英語表現

ベッドに食事台を置きます。

- ④ Let me incline your bed to 30 degrees, the best angle for your easy eating.

  ベッドを30度傾斜にしますね。一番食べやすい角度です。

- ⑤ I'll tie your bib on.

  胸当てをつけましょう。

- ⑥ In order not to choke your foods, let's say, "Pa, Pa, Pa, Ta, Ta, Ta, Ka, Ka, Ka, Ra, Ra, Ra".

  食べものが咽喉にひっかからないように「パパパ，タタタ，カカカ，ラララ」と言いましょう。

- ⑦ I'll raise your head a little and hold it while you eat.

  食べている間，頭を少し上げて支えます。

- ⑧ Draw your chin in order to avoid taking foods into the airway.

  食物が気道に入るのを防ぐために，顎を引いてください。

- ⑨ You seem to lose your appetite.

  食欲がないようですね。

- ⑩ Can you bring your spoon to your mouth?

  スプーンを口に持っていけますか？

- ⑪ You can handle chopsticks with springs very well.

  バネ付き箸の扱いが上手ですね。

- ⑫ Swallowing jerry is a good training for you to prevent accidental ingestion.

  ゼリーを飲み込むのは，誤嚥を起こさないためによい訓練です。

- ⑬ Minced meal often gets stuck in your throat.

  刻んだ食べ物は喉に詰まりやすいのです。

- ⑭ Chew your sponge cake well.

  スポンジケーキをよく噛んでください。

- ⑮ It will be easy for you to eat bread by tearing it off and dipping in milk.

  パンをちぎって，ミルクに浸すと食べやすいですよ。

- ⑯ Don't gobble up. You will choke.
  急いで食べないで。むせますから。
- ⑰ As you are on a restricted diet, you are not able to have another bowl of miso soup.
  食事が制限されていますので，味噌汁のお代わりはできないのです。

A. Before and after the meal　食前，食後

- ① Let's eat.
  Let's enjoy meal.
  いただきましょう。
- ② The food looks great!
  That looks very good!
  Looks yummy (delicious)!
  It sure smells good!
  おいしそうですね。
- ③ Are you satisfied?
  おわりましたか？
- ④ You ate up (polished off) food.
  すっかり食べましたね。
- ⑤ You seem to be [completely] full (stuffed).
  おなかがいっぱいになったようですね。
- ⑥ I hope you enjoyed the meal!
  おいしかったですか。
- ⑦ I'll clear the table.
  膳を下げましょう。

B. Taking medicine　薬の服用

- ① Take this medicine.
  この薬を飲んでください。

- ② Swallow this medicine, if you can.
  できれば，この薬を飲み込んでください。
- ③ This medicine should ease the pain.
  この薬は痛みを和らげます。

1-6. Grooming Activities　整容動作

- fix oneself up　身だしなみを整える
- wash (wipe) one's face　顔を洗う（拭く）
- rinse out one's mouth　口をすすぐ
- rinse out one's hands　水で手を洗う
- rinse off (out of ...; from ...)
  〔汚れ，石鹸，シャンプーなどを〕洗い流す
- brush one's teeth　歯磨きをする
- make up; put on make up　化粧する
- cut (pare; trim) one's nails　爪を切る

A. Hand-washing　手洗い

- ① Push the faucet with the back of your unaffected hand.
  水道の蛇口を患部でない方の手の甲で押してください。
- ② Can you move your wheelchair a little forward to under the washstand?
  車椅子を洗面台の下にもう少し動かせますか？
- ③ Lather some soap in your hands.
  手で石鹸を泡立てましょう。
- ④ Sit on the chair when you are tired, and rub your palms each other with soap bubbles.
  疲れたら椅子に座って，石鹸の泡で掌を両手でこすりあわせましょう。

- ☐ ⑤ This movement help you relax in order to get your stiff hands flexible.
  この動きはこわばった手を緩めリラックスさせます。
- ☐ ⑥ Movement in the form of a prayer is a good training to relax yourself.
  祈りの形の動きはリラックスするための良い訓練になります。
- ☐ ⑦ Open your fingers slowly and wash them completely.
  指の間もゆっくり開いてしっかり洗いましょう。
- ☐ ⑧ Rinse your hands out.
  手を洗い流しましょう。
- ☐ ⑨ Dry your hands off with air towel.
  エアタオルで両手を乾かしましょう。
- ☐ ⑩ Washing hands is very important not only for keeping you clean but [for] preventing from many diseases.
  手洗いは，清潔に保つだけでなく，多くの病気の予防のためにとても重要です。

B. Face-washing　洗顔

- ☐ ① Use this shallow basin when you wash your face.
  顔を洗うとき，この浅い洗面器を使いましょう。
- ☐ ② Are you reluctant to wash your face?
  顔を洗うのは気が進みませんか？
- ☐ ③ If so, you may only wipe your face with a wet towel.
  そうでしたら，濡れたタオルで顔を拭くだけでもいいですよ。
- ☐ ④ By covering the soaked towel on the faucet and squeezing it several times, you can make a wet towel easily.
  水に浸したタオルを蛇口にかけてねじると，簡単に濡れタオルができます。
- ☐ ⑤ Wipe the behind of your ears, because they tend to get dirty.
  耳の後ろも，汚れがたまりやすいので拭きましょう。

Part 4 **Useful Expressions for Rehabilitation** リハビリテーションに役立つ英語表現

C. Tooth-brushing　歯磨き

- ① The electric toothbrush is convenient but a little heavy for your weak fingers.
  電動歯ブラシは便利ですが，あなたの弱った指には少し重いでしょう。
- ② Let's move your toothbrush up and down but not from side to side, and brush the inside, too.
  歯ブラシを横ではなく上下に動かし，歯の裏側も磨きましょう。
- ③ Lift the cup with a holder to your mouth and rinse it out.
  ホルダー付きカップを口まで持ち上げ，よくすすぎましょう。
- ④ Wipe around your mouth with paper towel.
  口の周りをペーパータオルで拭きましょう。
- ⑤ Let's make it a rule to brush teeth after every meal.
  いつも食後に歯磨きをすることにしましょう。

D. Hair-washing　洗髪

- ① Rinse the shampoo out of your hair.
  シャンプーを洗い流しましょう。
- ② I'll fix a dryer, when you dry your hair.
  髪を乾かすときは，私がドライヤーを持ちます。
- ③ As the movement of your elbow joint is restricted, comb your hair with the brush with a long handle.
  ひじ関節の動きが制限されているので，長い柄のついたブラシで髪をとかしましょう。
- ④ In order to wash your hair on the bed, I will move your head close to the edge of the bed, and your legs to the opposite side.
  寝たままで洗髪するために，頭をベッドの端に近づけ，脚を頭の逆方向に動かします。
- ⑤ You may make an appointment with a hairdresser tomorrow.
  明日，美容室の予約を取れますよ。

E. Cutting nails 爪切り

- ① I'm afraid it's better to clip your nails.
  爪を切った方がよさそうです。
- ② Your nail is coming off.
  爪がはがれそうです。
- ③ I will help you cut them with a nail clippers attached with a board.
  板のついた爪切りで爪を切るのを手伝います。

F. Shaving / Making up ひげ剃り / 化粧

- ① You have been unshaven for these days.
  最近ひげを剃っていませんね。
- ② How about shaving by fixing an electric shaver to your hand?
  電気カミソリのブラシを手に固定して，ひげを剃るのはどうですか。
- ③ Lift your chin up a little.
  顎を少し上げてください。
- ④ You looked so nice when you make yourself up!
  お化粧するととてもきれいに見えますよ。
- ⑤ Fixing ourselves up everyday is good for our physical and mental health.
  毎日，身だしなみを整えるのは，心身にとってよいことです。

1-7. Bathing Activities 入浴動作

- take a shower シャワーを浴びる
- take a bath; enter the bath tub 入浴する
- turn on a hot tap お湯を出す
- wash oneself 身体を洗う
- rinse the soap off 石鹸を洗い流す
- dry oneself with a bath towel タオルで身体を拭く

Part 4 **Useful Expressions for Rehabilitation** リハビリテーションに役立つ英表現

- [ ] shampoo one's hair; wash one's hair　髪を洗う
- [ ] rinse off with warm water　髪をお湯で洗い流す
- [ ] dry one's hair with a towel　頭をタオルで拭く
- [ ] blow dry　ドライヤーで乾かす

- [ ] ① Let's try to take a bath by yourself.
  一人でお風呂に入ってみましょう。
- [ ] ② As you are difficult to raise your arm, wash your back with a back brush.
  腕が上がりにくいので，背中洗い用ブラシで背中を洗いましょう。
- [ ] ③ Let's enter the bathtub.
  湯船に入りましょう。
- [ ] ④ Sit on the bench beside the bathtub.
  バスタブの傍のベンチに座ってください。
- [ ] ⑤ Move your hips toward the bath tub slowly.
  腰をゆっくりとバスタブの方へ動かしてください。
- [ ] ⑥ First, put your right leg into the water.
  まず，右脚を湯に入れます。
- [ ] ⑦ I'll hold you until you completely enter the water.
  完全に湯に入るまで私が支えています。
- [ ] ⑧ Don't get in too deep.
  身体を深く沈めないでください。
- [ ] ⑨ How is the bath?
  湯加減はいかがですか？
- [ ] ⑩ Please let me know if the water is too hot or not warm enough.
  お湯が熱すぎたり，ぬるければ教えてください。
- [ ] ⑪ Please soak leisurely and relax.
  ゆったりと浸かってリラックスしてください。

- ☐ ⑫ If you feel ill or dizzy, just push the buzzer when I do not accompany you.
  私がいないときに気分が悪くなったり，眩暈がしたら，ブザーを押してください。
- ☐ ⑬ Please hold of the handrail when you get out of the bath not to slip and fell.
  お風呂から出るときは，すべって転げないように手すりをつかんでください。
- ☐ ⑭ You look a little tired, so shampoo your hair some other time.
  疲れているようですから，洗髪はまたの機会にしましょう。
- ☐ ⑮ We will help you take a bath in the caring bathtub as you are lying on the stretcher.
  寝たまま入浴できる介護浴槽でお風呂に入るお手伝いをします。

1-8. Toilet Activities 排泄動作

- ☐ pass urine; urinate; micturate　排尿する
- ☐ relieve oneself; make water; pass water; take a leak
  排尿する，トイレに行く《婉曲表現》
- ☐ piss　排尿する，小便する《俗語》
- ☐ piddle; pee; pee-pee; wee-wee; go number one
  排尿する，おしっこする《幼児語》
- ☐ defecate　排便する《専門》
- ☐ empty (evacuate; relieve; move) the bowels
  排便する，大便をする《婉曲表現》
- ☐ have a bowel movement
  排便する，便通（お通じ）がある
- ☐ poop; go number two　排便する，うんちをする《幼児語》

Part 4 **Useful Expressions for Rehabilitation** リハビリテーションに役立つ英語表現

- [ ] have (need) to go to the bathroom frequently
  トイレが近い
- [ ] flush the toilet　トイレの水を流す

- [ ] ① You haven't had a bowel movement for three days.
  3日間お通じがありません。
- [ ] ② You seem to have been constipated.
  便秘しているようですね。
- [ ] ③ Please sit on the toilet a little longer to have a bowel movement.
  便通があるように，少し長く便器に座ってみましょう。
- [ ] ④ I will move the wheelchair close to the toilet seat.
  車椅子を便座に近づけます。
- [ ] ⑤ I will help you get up on the bed and take a sitting position.
  ベッドに起き上がって座位をとりましょう。
- [ ] ⑥ Please stretch your back bone with my support.
  身体を支えますから，背骨を伸ばしましょう。
- [ ] ⑦ Sit on the portable toilet seat and shift yourself to the right direction.
  腰を右にずらして，ポータブル便座に座ってください。
- [ ] ⑧ Can you hold it to the toilet?
  トイレまで我慢できますか？
- [ ] ⑨ If you can't, I'm going to insert the bedpan.
  我慢できないなら，差し込み便器を入れますよ。
- [ ] ⑩ Stand up slowly as grasping the handrail.
  手すりを持って，ゆっくりと立ち上がります。
- [ ] ⑪ Never mind when you have toilet accidents.
  トイレの粗相をしても気にしないでください。

- ⑫ Press this call-button when you feel bad.
  気分が悪くなったら，このコールボタンを押してください。
- ⑬ Lack of exercise or dietary fiber and water, aging, light eating or some diseases may cause constipation.
  運動不足や食物繊維，水分の不足，加齢，少食，病気が，便秘の原因になる可能性があります。
- ⑭ We often need to go to the bathroom as we get old.
  歳をとるとトイレが近くなりがちです。
- ⑮ Let's exercise to strengthen the abdominal and back muscles.
  腹筋や背筋を強くする運動をしましょう。

1-9. Standard of Exercises for ADL
日常生活動作のための基本的運動

- go up and down the stairs　階段を昇り降りする
- take an elevator　エレベータを使う
- puff one's cheeks　頬を膨らませる
- rotate (turn around) the wrists　手首を回す
- bend one's neck back up　首をそらす
- crouch down　身体を丸める
- stretch one's back　背中をそらす
- straddle one's legs　両脚を広げる
- bend one's knees　膝を曲げる
- get on your knees　膝で立つ
- squat down　しゃがむ
- take a deep breath　深呼吸をする
- stride along with music　音楽に合わせて大股で歩く
- shuffle　足を引きずって歩く
- totter　よろめく
- trip over (on) ...　～につまずく

Part 4 **Useful Expressions for Rehabilitation**　リハビリテーションに役立つ英語表現

☐ land on your bum (backside; bottom)　しりもちをつく

A. Exercises anywhere　どこでもできる運動

☐ ① Let's try some simple exercises in the sitting position.
座った姿勢で簡単な運動をしてみましょう。

☐ ② Straighten and stretch your back, first.
まず背中をまっすぐに伸ばしてみましょう。

☐ ③ Puff out your cheeks.
頬を膨らませてください。

☐ ④ Open and close your mouth repeatedly.
口を開けたり閉じたり，繰り返してください。

☐ ⑤ Move your mouth (eyes) to the left and right repeatedly.
口（目）を左右に繰り返し動かしてください。

☐ ⑥ These exercises are effective in preventing muscular weakness around your mouth.
これらの運動は口の周りの筋肉が弱くなるのを防ぐのに効果的です。

☐ ⑦ Open your fingers as wide as possible and rotate the wrists.
指をできるだけ開いて，手首を回してください。

☐ ⑧ Count from one to ten on your fingers.
指で1から10まで数えてください。

☐ ⑨ Lie down on the floor (bed).
床（ベッド）に横になってください。

B. Basic exercises　基本運動

☐ ① Taking a right position is more essential than a walking activity.
正しい姿勢をとることは歩くよりももっと大切です。

☐ ② Do not over do. Just enjoy yourself in any position you are.
やりすぎないでください。どんな姿勢でもよいので楽しんでください。

- ③ Every activity in the daily life, for example, going to the toilet, the bathroom or going shopping, owes to walking.

  例えば，トイレや風呂場に行く，買物に出かける，というようなあらゆる日常生活での動作は，歩けるからできるのです。

- ④ Walking is essential for preventing your bedridden life, susceptibility of stumbling and bone fracture, depression and a decline in your will to live.

  歩くことは，寝たきり生活にならないように，またつまずいたり骨折したり，うつや生きる意欲の減退を防ぐのに必要不可欠です。

- ⑤ Various ADL activities are effective on functional recovery or maintenance of movement disorders such as joint contracture and paralysis of any part of your body.

  さまざまなADL動作は，身体のあらゆる部分の関節の硬直や麻痺のような運動障害に対して，機能回復や保持に有効です。

- ⑥ Let's go up stairs to your room, not taking an elevator.

  部屋までエレベータを使わないで，階段を昇りましょう。

- ⑦ Shall we take a rest when we reach at the landing?

  踊り場に着いたら休みましょうか？

- ⑧ Sitting down on the chair without leaning on the back is a good training for you to empty the bowels.

  椅子に背中をつけないで座ることは，排泄するための良い訓練です。

- ⑨ Sit on the chair (bed), and rub your knees slowly with feeling their roundness.

  椅子（ベッド）に座り，ひざを，その丸みを感じながら，ゆっくりこすってください。

- ⑩ Massage your hands or knees not only helps you relax but let the blood or lymph flow well.

  手やひざのマッサージは，リラックスさせるだけでなく，血液やリンパの流れをよくします。

Part 4 **Useful Expressions for Rehabilitation**　リハビリテーションに役立つ英語表現

1-10. Basic Training of Techniques for Occupational Therapy
　基礎作業療法

Art therapy	**芸術療法**
☐ Ceramics	陶芸
☐ rough wedging	荒練り(揉み)
☐ spiral wedging	菊練り
☐ forming with coils	紐作り
☐ biscuit firing	素焼き
☐ glazing	釉(くすり)がけ
☐ kiln; gaskiln; electric kiln	窯；ガス窯；電気窯
☐ **Leather work; leather craft/Cloisonné/ Wood carving** 革細工 / 七宝焼き / 木彫	
☐ chisel	のみ
☐ collage; torn-paper picture	コラージュ；ちぎり絵, 切り貼り絵
☐ glue; adhesive	接着剤
☐ handmade Japanese paper	和紙
☐ leather goods	革製品
☐ metalwork	金工
☐ mosaic work	モザイク細工
☐ plane	カンナ
☐ punching	刻印打ち
☐ swivel cutter; swivel cutting knife	スーベルカッター
☐ woodwork	木工
☐ **Painting**	**絵画**
☐ paint a picture	〔水彩画, 油絵を〕描く
☐ draw a picture	〔鉛筆, ペン, クレヨン画を〕描く
☐ appreciate pictures	絵画を鑑賞する
☐ **Calligraphy**	**書道**
☐ ink stone	硯

☐ Indian ink; Chinese ink	墨汁
☐ sumi; ink stick	固形の墨
☐ writing blush	毛筆
☐ **Haiku (poem); Japanese poem**	**俳句**
☐ write (compose) haiku	俳句を作る
☐ season word	季語
☐ punctuation words	切れ字
☐ **Music**	**音楽**
☐ mixed chorus	混声合唱
☐ ensemble	合奏
☐ musical performance	演奏
Miscellaneous	**その他**
☐ knitting	編み物
☐ macramé	マクラメ
☐ gardening	園芸
☐ garden products	園芸作物
☐ gardening tools	園芸用具

Ceramics 陶芸

☐ ① You told me you would like to try ceramic art the other day, didn't you?

先日，陶芸をしてみたいと言われましたね。

☐ ② Among rehabilitation medicine, ceramics or ceramic art has a long history as an occupational therapy.

陶芸はリハビリテーション医療の中で，作業療法の手段として古い歴史をもっています。

Part 4 **Useful Expressions for Rehabilitation**　リハビリテーションに役立つ英語表現

- ③ In the process of ceramic works from kneading clay to actual firing, you may feel a sense of unity with nature.
  粘土をこねることから本焼きまでの過程で，自然との一体感を覚えるかもしれません。
- ④ Well, with no further ado, let's start the first step, rough wedging.
  さて，講釈はこれくらいにして，最初の一歩の荒揉みを始めましょう。
- ⑤ Knead clay as shifting your weight on the palms.
  体重を手の平にかけて土を練ります。
- ⑥ Before you go to a next step, forming with coils, you need to mold a round bottom.
  次のステップの紐つくりに入る前に，丸い底を作っておきます。
- ⑦ Then, stretch clay to form a coil, and stick it to the bottom tightly with your fingers.
  そして粘土を伸ばして紐をつくり，しっかりと指で底につけます。
- ⑧ By piling up coils very carefully, what you want to make will be formed.
  紐を注意深く重ねることで，あなたが作りたいものが成形されます。
- ⑨ The remaining processes are drying, glazing, biscuit, and glost firing.
  残りの工程は，乾燥，釉薬，素焼き，本焼きです。
- ⑩ We are excited to see what a piece will come out!
  どんな作品ができるか楽しみですね！

2 Physical Exercises
身体運動

2-1. Basic Exercises 基本的運動

- [ ] be effective on ...　…に効果的である
- [ ] bend　（身体を）曲げる
- [ ] crouch down　うずくまる
- [ ] extend; stretch　（手足，身体を）伸展する，伸ばす
- [ ] flex　（手足，身体を）屈曲する，曲げる
- [ ] move (transfer) from A to B　AからBへ移動する
- [ ] place A on B　AをBに置く
- [ ] pinch up ...　…をつまみ上げる
- [ ] put a crutches under one's arms　腋の下に松葉杖を挟む
- [ ] raise oneself up　上半身を起こす
- [ ] relax ...　…を緩める
- [ ] relieve a pain　痛みを緩和する
- [ ] sit down with one's legs stretched　脚を伸ばして座る
- [ ] squat down　しゃがむ
- [ ] straddle one's legs　脚を拡げる
- [ ] stride along ...　…に合わせて大股で歩く
- [ ] take a deep breath　深呼吸をする

- [ ] ① Let's do some stretching for ten seconds to bend your body to either side.
  身体を左右に曲げるストレッチを10秒やりましょう。
- [ ] ② Bend your neck (upper body) forward, and back it up.
  首（上半身）を前方へ曲げ，それから後ろへそらしてください。
- [ ] ③ Lie on your back on the mat.
  マットに仰向けになってください。

Part 4 **Useful Expressions for Rehabilitation** リハビリテーションに役立つ英語表現

- ④ Move your legs as if you pedal a bicycle.
  自転車をこいでいるかのように脚を動かしてください。
- ⑤ Stand up beside the table, please.
  テーブルの横に立ってください。
- ⑥ Push the table top with each finger.
  テーブルの表面を1本1本の指で押してください。
- ⑦ Placing your hands on the table, repeat the motion of tapping.
  テーブルの上に両手を置き，指先でトントンする動作を繰り返してください。
- ⑧ In the same standing position, repeat the motion of crouching down and standing up.
  同じ立ち位置で，うずくまる，立つという動作を繰り返してください。
- ⑨ Straddle your legs a little and stretch your arms as high as possible.
  両脚を少し広げて，両腕をできるだけ高く伸ばしてください。
- ⑩ Make a big circle with your arms at the shoulder joint.
  肩の関節の位置で大きく両腕を回しましょう。
- ⑪ Imagine you are making a very big pancake around your shoulders.
  肩のあたりで巨大なパンケーキを作っていると想像してみてください。
- ⑫ Let's stride along as swinging your arms with music.
  両腕を音楽に合わせて揺らしながら大股で歩きましょう。
- ⑬ Now, take a deep breath.
  深呼吸をします。

2-2. Basic Range of Motion (ROM) Exercise 基本的可動域運動

A. Exercise of joints 関節の運動

- Active movement of ankle joints
  足関節と足部の自動運動

☐ ① Place your leg on the sloped cushion in the dorsal position.
  仰臥位で脚をクッションに載せてください。

☐ ② Flex your affected foot toward yourself.
  患側の足をあなたの方に曲げてください。

☐ ③ Then, extend it toward the bed.
  そしてベッドの方に伸ばしてください。

☐ ④ This exercise is effective against edema and deep vein thrombosis after operation.
  この運動は手術後の浮腫と深部静脈血栓症に効果的です。

- Self assistive active movement of knee joint
  膝関節の自己介助自動運動

☐ ① Sit down with your legs stretched on the mat.
  マットに脚を伸ばして腰を降ろしてください。

☐ ② Place one of your hands just below the knee, and the other on the lower part of the leg.
  片方の手を膝の下に，もう一方を脚の下の方に，置いてください。

☐ ③ Flex your knee, tying to draw it toward your chest.
  膝を曲げて，胸の方に引き寄せてみてください。

☐ ④ This exercise will relieve a pain you have in the early period after operation of your knee joint.
  この運動は，膝関節の手術後早い時期に感じる痛みを緩和します。

Part 4 **Useful Expressions for Rehabilitation** リハビリテーションに役立つ英語表現

- Active assistive movement for knee joint
  膝関節の自動介助的運動

☐ ① Lie on your back.
  仰向けに寝てください。

☐ ② Let me put your lower leg on my leg and hold your foot under my arm.
  あなたの下腿を私の足の上にのせ，腕の下で足を支えます。

☐ ③ I'll help you bend the knee by pressing it.
  私が膝を押して，あなたが膝を曲げるのを手伝います。

☐ ④ At the same time, I will push your calf toward the knee.
  同時に，ふくらはぎを膝の方に向けて押します。

☐ ⑤ Imagine you are drawing your thigh toward the stomach.
  太ももをお腹に引き寄せていると想像してください。

B. Stretching ストレッチング

- Stretching of Achilles tendon and triceps muscle of calf
  アキレス腱，下腿三頭筋のストレッチング

☐ ① Stand in front of the wall, taking a step forward.
  壁の前に立って一歩前に出ます。

☐ ② Put your hands on the wall.
  両手を壁につけます。

☐ ③ Keeping heels on the floor, lean forward as you shift your weight forth.
  かかとは床につけたまま，体重を前にかけながら前方へ傾けます。

☐ ④ Also you should not move your buttocks backward.
  またお尻も後ろに動かさないでください。

☐ ⑤ This exercise gets both of the Achilles tendon and the triceps [muscle] of calf stretched.
  この運動は，アキレス腱と下腿三頭筋を伸ばしてくれます。

- Stretching for hamstring　ハムストリングのストレッチング

☐ ① Sit on the floor with your legs extended.
　　両脚を伸ばして床に座ってください。

☐ ② Bend your upper body and hold your toes.
　　上半身を前に倒してつま先を持ちます。

☐ ③ Then raise yourself up.
　　そして上半身を元に戻します。

☐ ④ Repeat this exercise several times.
　　この運動を何回か繰り返します。

☐ ⑤ This movement will increase flexibility of your leg muscles and prevent a rupture of the hamstring.
　　この動きは，あなたの脚の筋肉の柔軟性を高め，ハムストリングの断裂を防ぎます。

C. Muscle-strengthening exercise　筋力増強運動

- Squatting movement　スクワット運動

☐ ① Have an upright position in front of the bar, or between two bars.
　　バーの前，または2本のバーの間で直立の姿勢をとります。

☐ ② Squat down and stand up repeatedly at a slow speed with catching the bar.
　　バーをつかんだまま，ゆっくりとかがんだり，立ったりします。

☐ ③ This exercise will strengthen your quadriceps [muscle] of thigh with its centrifugal contraction.
　　この運動は，遠心性収縮で，大腿四頭筋を強くします。

☐ ④ You can do this exercise with putting hands on a table at your home as well.
　　この運動は，あなたの家でも，テーブルに手を置いてできます。

Part 4 **Useful Expressions for Rehabilitation** リハビリテーションに役立つ英語表現

- Muscle-strengthening exercise for the affected and unaffected upper limbs　患側・健側の上肢筋力増強運動

☐ ① Sit on the stool.
　　丸椅子に座ってください。

☐ ② Hold one of the hoops with your affected hand.
　　患側の手で1つ輪を持ってください。

☐ ③ Stretch your hand and pull the hoop down slowly.
　　その手を伸ばして，輪をゆっくり引っぱり降ろします。

☐ ④ You can put a loading weight to the other hoop for additional resistance on the healthy side.
　　健側に抵抗を与えるために一方の輪に負荷を加えてもかまいません。

☐ ⑤ This movement will strengthen both of your affected and healthy upper limbs.
　　この運動は，患側と健側の両方の上肢を強くします。

D. Strengthening abdominal muscles　腹筋の強化

☐ ① Lie on your back on the mat with your arms crossed in front of the chest.
　　マットに仰向けになり，胸の前で腕を組んでください。

☐ ② Bend your knees and raise your upper body.
　　膝を曲げて上半身を起こします。

☐ ③ This exercise in the flexed the position of the hip joint will strengthen your abdominal muscles.
　　股関節屈曲位でのこの運動は，あなたの腹筋を強くします。

E. Exercise of resistive movement　抵抗運動

- Movement of upper limbs　上肢の運動

☐ ① Sit down on the chair.
　　椅子に座ってください。

- ☐ ② I'll put a weight on your wrist for additional load.
  手首にさらに負荷をかけるために重りをつけます。
- ☐ ③ Raise your hand and extend it slowly.
  手を上げてゆっくり伸ばします。

- Movement of lower limbs　下肢の運動
- ☐ ① Let me pass an elastic band through each of your lower legs.
  両方の下腿にゴムの輪をかけます。
- ☐ ② I'll twist it (an elastic band) between your ankles.
  両足首のところで（ゴムを）ねじります。
- ☐ ③ Pull and relax it (an elastic band) as many times as possible.
  できるかぎり繰り返し，ゴムを引っぱり，ゆるめます。
- ☐ ④ This is a resistive exercise of the quadriceps [muscle] of the thigh as well as the gluteus [muscle].
  これは，大腿四頭筋と中殿筋の抵抗運動です。
- ☐ ⑤ If you have any disorder in the hip joint when strengthening the gluteus [muscle], you can put a shorter band above the knee.
  And so, that will prevent too much pressure on the knee.
  中殿筋強化のとき，股関節に障害があるなら，膝の上に短いバンドを付けます。そうすると膝に圧力がかかりすぎるのを防げます。

F. Walking, going up and down stairs, transferring 歩行, 階段昇降, 移乗

- Crutch gait　松葉杖を使用しての歩行
- ☐ ① Let's begin a walking exercise to prevent disuse atrophy after operation.
  手術後の廃用性萎縮を予防するために歩く練習を始めましょう。

Part 4 **Useful Expressions for Rehabilitation** リハビリテーションに役立つ英語表現

- ② Walking with a cane or crutches reduces the load on your joints.
  杖や松葉杖を使用して歩くと関節への負担が減ります。
- ③ I'll explain how to use crutches.
  松葉杖の使い方を説明します。
- ④ Put crutches under your armpits.
  松葉杖を腋の下に置きます。
- ⑤ Don't open your arms so wide.
  腕はあまり広げないでください。
- ⑥ And try to walk with as long strides as possible.
  そして，できるだけ大股で歩くようにしてください。
- ⑦ Don't worry. I'll walk together beside you.
  心配いりません。隣で一緒に歩きます。

- Going upstairs　階段を昇る
- ① When you go upstairs depending on crutches, put the healthy leg on the stairs first.
  松葉杖をつきながら階段を昇るときは，健側の足を先に出します。
- ② Then lift the affected leg on the stair together with crutches.
  それから，患側の足を松葉杖と一緒に出します。

- Going downstairs　階段を降りる
- ① When you go downstairs, place the affected leg together with crutches.
  階段を降りるときは，患側の足を松葉杖と一緒に出します。
- ② And put the unaffected leg down on the stair.
  それから，健側の足を降ろします。

- Hemiplegic patient's transfer movement
片麻痺患者の移乗動作

☐ ① When you move from the wheelchair to the bed, move the sliding (transfer) board on your affected side.
車椅子からベッドに移るときは，スライディングボードを患側に置いてください。

☐ ② You need to place your wheelchair diagonally to the bed.
車椅子をベッドの対角線上に置く必要があります。

☐ ③ While you are transferring, I'll hold your ankle in a cast to avoid its hitting the foot plate.
移動するとき，ギブスをはめている足首が踏み板にあたらないように，私が持ちます。

2-3. Manual Dexterity Exercises of Fingers 手指巧緻性訓練
Exercises with pegboard ペグボード訓練

☐ ① Putting pegs into the holes on the board is a very good exercise to recover your failure in coordination of voluntary muscular movement.
ボードの穴にペグをはめるのは，随意筋運動の協調の低下を回復するためにとても良い運動です。

☐ ② Among various kinds of peg board, we choose a little big pegs today.
いろいろな種類のペグボードの中で，今日は，少し大きいペグを選びます。

☐ ③ The exercise is also very simple and limited to permitted extent.
練習も単純で，許可された範囲に制限されます。

☐ ④ Pinch up a coloring peg between your thumb and any other finger of your affected side and put it into any hole on the board.

Part 4 **Useful Expressions for Rehabilitation** リハビリテーションに役立つ英語表現

患側の親指とほかのいずれかの指で色ペグをつまみ，ボードの穴に入れてください。

☐ ⑤ You are getting good at pinching pegs. Let's count how many pegs you could move.
ペグをつまむのが上手になりました。移動できたペグの数を数えましょう。

☐ ⑥ I'm afraid you are bored of the very simple activity, I mean, just transferring pegs from one side to the other.
ペグを一方側から別の側に移動するという，とても単純な運動に飽きたのではないかと思います。

☐ ⑦ If possible, how about describing a kind of design on the board with pegs?
できるならば，ペグで何かのデザインをボードに描いてはどうでしょう？

☐ ⑧ You may enjoy playing a match game on the board with your acquaintance.
知り合いの方とボードでマッチゲームを楽しめます。

☐ ⑨ Red-colored pegs belong to you, and blue ones to another, for example, a patient here.
赤のペグはあなたのもので，青が他の人，例えば，ここの患者さんのものです。

☐ ⑩ To recover the delicate movements of your stiffened fingers, you can choose other activities, such as building blocks, putting a jigsaw puzzle, bagging, passing strings through the holes or origami (paper folding) are also recommended.
以前のこわばった指の細かい動きを取り戻すために，他にもブロック重ね，ジグソーパズル，袋詰め，穴への糸通しや折紙などもお勧めします。

3 Rehabilitation for Diseases
疾患別リハビリテーション

3-1. Diseases of Locomotive Organs　運動器疾患

- [ ] expand the range of motion of ...
  …の関節可動域を拡げる
- [ ] fix by plaster　ギプスで固定する
- [ ] extend one's knee　膝を伸ばす(伸展する)
- [ ] get the hang in ...　…のコツを覚える
- [ ] grasp ...　…を握る
- [ ] have pain in ...　…に痛みがある
- [ ] lie on one's back　仰向けになる
- [ ] lie on one's stomach　うつぶせになる
- [ ] loosen ...　…を緩める
- [ ] pedal a bicycle　自転車をこぐ
- [ ] puff one's stomach　お腹を膨らませる
- [ ] prevent A from B　BからAを防ぐ
- [ ] put (place) A on B　Bの上にAを置く
- [ ] rotate one's hand　手を回す
- [ ] start rehab　リハビリを始める
- [ ] stretch one's leg　脚を伸ばす

A. Fracture　骨折
- Finger fracture　指骨骨折

- [ ] ① You're already free from pain caused from operation.
  手術の痛みは，もうないですね。
- [ ] ② Let's begin active exercise to prevent contracture of your fingers.
  指の拘縮を防ぐ自動運動を始めましょう。

Part 4 **Useful Expressions for Rehabilitation** リハビリテーションに役立つ英語表現

- ③ Put your affected hand on the pillow on the table.
  患側の手をテーブルの上の枕に置いてください。
- ④ Grasp a dumbbell in the wrist extension position.
  ダンベルを手首の伸展位で握ります。
- ⑤ Turn the wrist inward and outward by using the power of the dumbbell.
  ダンベルの力を利用しながら手首を内側と外側に回します。
- ⑥ Please remember to exercise at a moderate pace.
  適度なペースでやることを覚えておきましょう。
- ⑦ Excessive exercise will result in weaker muscular strength.
  運動をしすぎると結果的に筋力が弱くなります。

- Distal radius fracture　橈骨遠位端骨折
- ① Please extend your wrist.
  手首を伸ばしましょう。
- ② Flex your wrist downward with a slightly round-shaped hand.
  手を少し丸めた形で手首を下方に曲げてください。
- ③ Next, open all the fingers and flex the wrist upward.
  次に，指全部を広げ手首を上方に曲げてください。
- ④ Relax, and try not to bend and extend fingers too hard.
  リラックスして，あまり力まないで指を曲げたり伸ばしたりしましょう。
- ⑤ This exercise effects on keeping stability of the wrist joint fixing tenodesis action.
  この運動は腱を固定して，手首の安定に効果があります。

- Femoral diaphyseal fracture　大腿骨骨幹部骨折
- ① Lie on your back.
  仰向けになってください。

- ② I will place a weight on your stomach.
  おなかの上に重りを載せます。
- ③ Puff your stomach out and pull it in, so the weight goes up and down.
  お腹を膨らませ，引っ込めてください。すると重りが上下します。
- ④ Repeat this movement to strengthen the weak abdominal muscles.
  この動きを繰り返すことで弱い腹筋を強化します。

- Femoral neck fracture　大腿骨頚部骨折
  Before operation　術前
- ① I'll let you wear a weight on the lower part of your leg.
  脚の下部に重りを装着させます。
- ② I'll also place a cushion under your knees.
  膝の下にクッションを置きます。
- ③ Press down the cushion with your knees, and bend your feet with the weight on upward and extend them.
  クッションを膝で押し，重りをつけたまま足を上方へ曲げたり伸ばしたりします。
- ④ I'm sure this exercise is simple and easy for you staying in bed for a period of time.
  この運動は，きっとしばらく安静にしておられるあなたには単純で簡単にできると思います。
- ⑤ This muscular training also improves femoral neck fracture.
  これらの筋肉訓練は，大腿骨頚部骨折も改善します。

After operation　術後
- Standing up to sitting exercise　起立着座運動
- ① It's about time for you to start whole body exercise to prevent your body from disuse atrophy.

Part 4 **Useful Expressions for Rehabilitation** リハビリテーションに役立つ英語表現

身体を廃用性萎縮から予防するために全身の運動をそろそろ始めましょう。

☐ ② Let's raise your body to a standing position from the bed and sit down on it.
ベッドから身体を起して立ち上がり，ベッドの上に腰かけてください。

☐ ③ Oh, you are unsteady on your feet.
立ち上がると，不安定ですね。

☐ ④ When the forward-bending is not enough, you tend to land on your rear.
前屈姿勢が不十分だと，尻もちをつきやすくなります。

☐ ⑤ I prepared a reciprocal walker for you to support your standing.
立っているのを支えるために交互歩行器を準備しました。

☐ ⑥ You should repeat this standing-up movement very slowly.
この立ち上がり運動をとてもゆっくりと繰り返しましょう。

- Patellar fracture　膝蓋骨・骨折

☐ ① Lie on your stomach on the bed.
ベッドにうつぶせになってください。

☐ ② I'll put a weight on your ankle on the side of the fractured patella (knee cap).
骨折した膝蓋骨の方の足首に重りを載せます。

☐ ③ Lift up your leg and extend it slowly.
脚を上げてゆっくり伸ばしてください。

☐ ④ A weight adds resistance to the quadriceps [muscle] of thigh.
重りによって腿（もも）の大腿四頭筋へ抵抗が加わります。

☐ ⑤ When lifting your leg, stop at the appropriate angle to the bed.
脚を上げたら，ベッドに対して適当な角度で止めてください。

- ⑥ I mean, you must not stretch out the muscle too much.
  つまり，筋肉を伸ばしすぎないということです。

- Osteoporotic spinal compression fracture
  骨粗鬆症性脊椎圧迫骨折

Before giving physical therapy 理学療法の前に

- ① The cause of your lower back pain is osteoporosis.
  あなたが患っている腰痛の原因は，骨粗鬆症です。
- ② You have already worn soft corset (lumbosacral corset) since you broke the lower backbone.
  腰骨を折ってから既に，腰部コルセットを着けていますね。
- ③ It helps you to keep the lumbar stable.
  それは腰部を安定させるのに役立ちます。
- ④ Not to get disuse syndrome, you need to have physical therapy as early as possible.
  廃用症候群にならないように，できるだけ早く理学療法を受ける必要があります。
- ⑤ Elderly patients very likely do not exercise such rehabilitations as bridging or strengthening of lower limb muscles.
  高齢の患者さんは，きっとブリッジ運動や下肢の筋肉を伸ばすリハビリをしたがらないでしょう。
- ⑥ I'll introduce some exercises you can do by yourself.
  自分でできる運動をいくつか紹介します。

Exercise of the forward-bent movement 体幹前傾運動

- ① Sit down on the chair and spread out your legs.
  椅子に座って，脚を開いてください。
- ② Put your arms into the slings in front of you.
  両腕をあなたの前のスリングに入れてください。

Part 4 **Useful Expressions for Rehabilitation** リハビリテーションに役立つ英語表現

- ③ Move your trunk forward and backward and set a moving sling back to the original position.
  体幹を前後に動かし，動くスリングを元の位置まで戻します。
- ④ By this forward and backward bending motion of the trunk, the muscles of your back will get stretched and stronger.
  このように前後に体幹を曲げる運動は，腰の筋肉を伸ばして強くします。
- ⑤ You can do the same exercise by moving a big rubber ball.
  大きなゴムボールを動かすことでも同じ運動ができます。

B. Muscular injuries / Tendon injuries　筋損傷 / 腱損傷

- Finger flexor injuries　手指屈筋腱損傷
- ① The surgery went well, so let's start rehab a week later.
  手術はうまくいったので，1週間後からリハビリを始めましょう。
- ② Put your hand on the table.
  手を台の上に置いてください。
- ③ Bend your fingers and let your hand make a round shape.
  指を折り，手を丸い形にしてみましょう。
- ④ Stretch them out very slowly.
  指をゆっくり伸ばしてみましょう。
- ⑤ These active bending and stretching exercises of the fingers prevent their edema as well as contracture.
  このような指の自動屈伸運動は，浮腫と拘縮を防ぎます。

- Achilles tendon rupture　アキレス腱断裂
  Towel gathering exercise　タオルギャザリング
- ① Your lower leg has been fixed by plaster to protect ruptured Achilles tendon.
  下腿は，断裂したアキレス腱を守るためのギプスで固定されています。

☐ ② But you can pinch and haul in a towel on the floor with your toes sticking out.
   しかし，床の上でつま先を突き出して，タオルをつまんで引きよせることができます。
☐ ③ Towel gathering exercise is intended to keep the muscle strength of soles and toes.
   タオルギャザリング運動は，足裏とつま先の筋力を保つためのものです。
☐ ④ You will be able to do this simple exercise anywhere and anytime in the sitting position or standing one.
   この簡単な運動は，いつでもどこでも，座った姿勢でも立った姿勢でもできます。
☐ ⑤ Keep up your spirits! They say, "Where there is a will, there is a way."
   元気を出しましょう。「意志あるところに道あり」と言いますから。

Pedaling a stationary bicycle　固定自転車のペダル踏み

☐ ① When you have pain anywhere in the leg in plaster, you can prefer another exercise, for example, pedaling a stationary cycle.
   ギプスをしている脚のどこかに痛みがあるときは，別の運動，例えば，固定自転車のペダル踏みがよいでしょう。
☐ ② Sit on the bicycle-ergometer.
   自転車エルゴメーターに座ります。
☐ ③ Hold the bar and pedal it slowly.
   バーをつかんでゆっくりこぎます。
☐ ④ Ergometer, an apparatus on a stationary bicycle, is used to measure the muscle power during your physical exercise.
   エルゴメーターは，固定自転車の装置ですが，運動中の筋力の測定に使われます。

Part 4 **Useful Expressions for Rehabilitation** リハビリテーションに役立つ英語表現

☐ ⑤ This movement is also effective in strengthening muscles of your lower limbs.
　この運動は，下肢の筋力強化にも効果的です。

C. Arthritis　関節炎

- Scapulohumeral periarthiritis　肩関節周囲炎

☐ ① Put your affected forearm on the table fixing it close to the side of your body.
　患側の前腕をテーブルに置いて身体の横につけてください。

☐ ② Rotate your hand to the right and left without shifting your shoulder blade.
　肩甲骨を動かさずに手を左右に回します。

☐ ③ This exercise trains infraspinatus, teres minor muscle and subscapular muscle.
　この運動は，棘下筋，小円筋，そして肩甲骨下筋を鍛えます。

☐ ④ If you have any pain, please let me know.
　痛みがあるときには教えてください。

☐ ⑤ We will provide you a device for recovering the muscular strength in the state where pains are eased.
　痛みが和らげられた状態で筋力を回復させる装具を用意します。

- Hip osteoarthritis　変形性股関節症

☐ ① Lie on your back on the mat.
　マットの上に仰向けになってください。

☐ ② I will press your right knee as it is extended.
　右膝を伸ばしたまま押さえます。

☐ ③ Then, I'll bend the knee close to your stomach.
　そして膝をお腹に向かって曲げます。

☐ ④ Next, I'll do the same movement on the other leg.
　次に，もう一方の脚にも同じ動きをします。

- ☐ ⑤ Please put up with pain as much as you can.
　できるだけ痛みは我慢してください。
- ☐ ⑥ This stretching exercise is intended to maintain and expand the range of motion of the muscles of your hip joints.
　このストレッチ運動は，股関節の筋肉の可動域を維持し拡張するためのものです。
- ☐ ⑦ Repeat this [stretching] movement ten times on each leg everyday.
　この〔ストレッチ〕運動を10回それぞれの脚に毎日繰り返します。

D. Inversion strain of ankle joint　足関節内反捻挫
- Exercise of strengthening fibular muscle　腓骨筋強化訓練

- ☐ ① A month has passed since you strained the ankle joint, and you are able to walk without pain now.
　足首を捻挫して以来1ヵ月経過して，今は痛みなく歩けますよ。
- ☐ ② But you need some exercise to make your peroneal muscles strong, not to have a further inversion strain of the ankle joint.
　でも，さらに足関節内反捻挫を起こさないように，腓骨筋を強くする練習が必要です。
- ☐ ③ Put your foot into the loop tied to the pole.
　柱にくくったひもの輪に足を入れてください。
- ☐ ④ Pull it (the loop) outward.
　それを足で外側へ引っ張ってください。
- ☐ ⑤ Now loosen it (the loop).
　次に緩めましょう。
- ☐ ⑥ Repeat this exercise as many times as you can.
　この練習をできるかぎり何度も反復してください。
- ☐ ⑦ You can also stretch the lower leg any time at your home.
　下腿のストレッチは自宅でいつでもできます。

Part 4 **Useful Expressions for Rehabilitation**　リハビリテーションに役立つ英語表現

E. Amputation　切断

① I understand the loss of your dominant hand is the bitter fact, but let's train and acquire some movements with your artificial hand from now on.
利き手をなくしてしまわれてお辛いと思いますが，これから義手でできる運動を覚えて，身につけましょう。

② Before training, you have to exercise enough the range of motion and muscles of the upper limbs, such as the girdle and the shoulder or the elbow joint.
訓練を始める前に，上肢の肩甲帯，肩関節，肘関節などの可動域運動と筋力を強める運動を十分しておきましょう。

③ Next, don't forget to rock the part of the elbow of the harness to control its power automatically.
次に，肘の部分をロックすることを忘れないで，ハーネスの力をコントロールするコツを身体で覚えます。

④ Now, let's train opening and closing motions of the artificial hand.
それでは，義手の開閉の訓練をしましょう。

⑤ We prepare some daily goods, for example, blocks for piling up exercise, and small soft and hard balls for pinching.
いくつかの日常品を用意しています。例えば，積み上げ練習用のブロックやつまみ練習用の軟らかい玉と硬い玉などです。

⑥ Will you prefer pinch activity? It might be simple but difficult to do with your artificial hand.
つまみ動作をしましょうか？ 単純ですが，義手でするのは難しいかもしれません。

⑦ Please pinch a soft ball in the box and put it in the other empty box by opening and closing your [artificial] hand.
義手を開閉して箱の中にある柔らかい玉をつまみ，空の箱に入れてください。

- ⑧ Take it easy. Oh, you are getting the hang in pinching.
  ゆっくりしましょう。ピンチ動作のコツを覚えてきましたね。
- ⑨ You are good at pinching soft balls. Let's do the same training with hard ones.
  やわらかい玉を挟むのは上手になりました。次は，硬い玉で同じ訓練をしましょう。
- ⑩ You lost your dominant hand, but writing letters is necessary in your daily life.
  利き手をなくされましたが，文字を書くのは日常生活で必要なことです。
- ⑪ Let's begin writing training with the left hand little by little from now on.
  これから少しずつ左手で書字訓練を始めましょう。

F. Lower back pain　腰痛

- ① Get on all fours on the floor.
  床に両手両足をつけてください。
- ② Raise one of your hands and the leg of the opposite side as high as possible.
  一方の手とその反対側の脚をできるだけ高く上げてください。
- ③ Repeat the same exercise with the other hand and leg.
  同じ運動を反対側の手と脚で繰り返します。
- ④ With this exercise, you'll produce the rotation of the pelvic bone and prevent hyperextension of the lumbar vertebrae.
  この運動で，骨盤の回転を生じ，腰椎の過伸展を予防します。

- Acute back bone pain　急性腰痛症
- ① Please stay in bed when you have severe pain.
  ひどい痛みがあるときはベッドに横になっていてください。

Part 4 **Useful Expressions for Rehabilitation**　リハビリテーションに役立つ英語表現

- ② I'll put a pillow under your knees, and a folded towel under your waist to keep your functional position.
  膝の下に枕を，腰の下にはたたんだタオルを入れて機能的位置を保ちます。
- ③ Do you still have pain in your lower back? No?
  腰にまだ痛みがありますか。ありませんか。
- ④ That's because the inflammation has calmed and the pain has disappeared.
  炎症が治まって痛みがなくなったのです。

- Mackenzie exercise　マッケンジー体操（腰痛体操）

- ① Your lumbar vertebrae curves a little in the abdominal (prone) position.
  腰椎が腹臥位になって少し曲がっています。
- ② Well, will you start Mackenzie exercise?
  では，マッケンジー体操を始めましょう。
- ③ Lie down on your stomach, first.
  まず，腹ばいになってください。
- ④ Please keep the position for five to ten minutes.
  その姿勢を5〜10分保ってください。
- ⑤ If you have pain, let me know. I'll put a cushion under your stomach to keep the position as long as possible.
  痛みがあれば教えてください。クッションをお腹の下に入れてできるだけその姿勢が保てるようにします。
- ⑥ If you have no pain, bend your elbows to 90 degrees.
  痛みがなければ，肘を90度に曲げてください。
- ⑦ This posture makes the curve of your backbone large.
  この姿勢は，腰のそりを大きくします。
- ⑧ Keep this posture like the Sphinx for five to ten minutes.
  スフィンクスのようにこの姿勢を5〜10分保ちます。

- ☐ ⑨ If your hips or legs ache, do not continue the exercise. If you are all right, go ahead to the next exercise.
  もし腰や脚が痛くなったらこの運動を続けないでください。大丈夫なら，次に運動に進んでください。
- ☐ ⑩ Extend your arms and raise your upper body.
  両腕を伸ばして上半身を上げます。
- ☐ ⑪ While extending the body, please relax without using muscles of the back.
  身体を伸ばしている間，背中の筋肉を使わないでリラックスしてください。
- ☐ ⑫ Breathe enough and lower your abdomen toward the mat.
  十分息をして，お腹をマットの方へ下げていきます。
- ☐ ⑬ At the first or second time, you need to do these exercises very carefully.
  最初の1・2回は，これらの運動をとても注意深くやらなくてはいけません。
- ☐ ⑭ When you are all right, please go on the exercise every two or three hours.
  大丈夫なら，2～3時間ごとに運動を続けてください。
- ☐ ⑮ According to the improvement of the symptom, do the exercise four times a day.
  （腰の）症状が改善されれば，1日4回この運動をしてください。

3-2. Cerebrovascular Accidents　脳血管障害

- ☐ add resistance to one's knee　膝に抵抗を加える
- ☐ assist sb to turn over　人が寝がえりするのを助ける
- ☐ avoid accidental ingestion　誤嚥を防ぐ
- ☐ bend (flex) one's knee to 90 degree
  膝を90度曲げる（屈曲する）

Part 4 **Useful Expressions for Rehabilitation** リハビリテーションに役立つ英語表現

- [ ] breathe in / out 息を吸う / 吐く
- [ ] breathe out with one's mouth pursed
  口をすぼめて息を吐く
- [ ] cross one's arms 腕を交差させる
- [ ] do pressure elimination 除圧動作をする
- [ ] do a warm up exercise 準備運動をする
- [ ] get bedsore 褥瘡になる
- [ ] help *sb* sit down 人が座るのを手伝う
- [ ] hold one's breath 息を止める
- [ ] lift one's buttocks up お尻を上げる
- [ ] perform the range of motion exercise
  関節可動域運動をする
- [ ] prevent contracture 拘縮を防ぐ
- [ ] put on a brace 装具を着ける
- [ ] put one's weight on ... …に重心をかける
- [ ] raise oneself 身体を起こす

A. Activity of turning over　寝がえり動作

- [ ] ① Raising yourself in the bed is a step to your daily life.
  ベッド上で身体を起こすことは日常生活への第一歩です。
- [ ] ② I'll assist you to turn over on the bed today.
  今日はベッドで寝がえりするお手伝いをします。
- [ ] ③ I'll bend your knees, and cross your arms on the chest.
  あなたの膝を曲げ，腕を胸で交差させます。
- [ ] ④ As the left half of your body is paralyzed, I'll stand on your right side.
  左半身が麻痺しているので，私は右側に立ちます。
- [ ] ⑤ Raise your head to me.
  頭を私の方に上げてください。

- ☐ ⑥ Let me insert my hand under your neck, and hold your hip.
  手をあなたの首の下に入れて，腰を支えます。
- ☐ ⑦ Then, I'll turn your body toward me with my hands.
  それから身体を私の方に両手で動かします。

B. Activity of self-lifting　起き上がり動作

- ☐ ① First, lift your affected arm supporting with the other unaffected one and join both hands.
  まず，患側の腕をもう一方の健側の手で支えながら持ち上げて，手を一緒に組んでください。
- ☐ ② Bend the knee on the unaffected side, and put it under the knee on the affected side.
  健側の膝を曲げて，患側の膝の下に入れてください。
- ☐ ③ Rest your elbow about 60 degrees apart from the body, and get up with it as the fulcrum.
  肘を身体から60度離してつき，振り子のようにして起きあがります。
- ☐ ④ Then, I'll take down your foot at the edge of the bed.
  次に，私があなたの足をベッドの端に降ろします。

C. Activity of standing up　立ち上がり動作

- ☐ ① Let's sit up in your bed.
  ベッドから起き上がりましょう。
- ☐ ② I'll help you to sit down on the edge of the bed.
  ベッドの端に座るのを私が手伝います。
- ☐ ③ Please bend your knees to nearly 90 degrees.
  両膝をほぼ90度に曲げてください。
- ☐ ④ Try to lift your buttocks up with your hands on the bed, and stoop to put your weight on your tiptoes.
  ベッドに両手をついてお尻を持ち上げ，つま先の方へ重心をかけるようにかがみます。

Part 4 **Useful Expressions for Rehabilitation** リハビリテーションに役立つ英語表現

☐ ⑤ When it is difficult for you to stand up, please put your hand on a nearby table.
立ち上がるのが難しいときは，近くのテーブルに手をついてください。

☐ ⑥ Then, stretch your legs. Well done, well done!
それから，脚を伸ばします。上手です，よくできましたね。

D. Walking exercises　歩行練習

☐ ① The paralysis of your left leg is not so serious.
左脚の麻痺はそれほどひどくありません。

☐ ② Let's put on short leg brace and start an exercise of walking.
短下肢装具を着けて歩く練習を始めましょう。

☐ ③ The brace will protect the back-knee of your paralyzed leg.
装具は麻痺した脚の膝の裏を守ります。

☐ ④ Hold the bar to ease your difficulty in walking.
バーを持って楽に歩いてみましょう。

☐ ⑤ Take your time. I'll walk with you.
ゆっくりやりましょう。私が一緒に歩きます。

E. Functional training of the upper limb　上肢機能訓練

☐ ① Hold a ball with your hands.
ボールを両手で握ってください。

☐ ② Extend your arms forward as holding the ball.
ボールを握りながら，両腕を前に伸ばします。

☐ ③ Then, bend your elbows and bring the ball close to your chest again.
それから，肘を曲げてボールをまた胸につけるように持ってきます。

☐ ④ Repeat this movement as often as possible.
できるだけ多くこの動きを繰り返します。

F. Facilitation to the adduction of the hip joint muscle　股関節内転筋促進

- ① Lie on your back.
  仰向けに横になってください。
- ② Let me pull your healthy leg outward.
  健側の足を外側に引っ張りますね。
- ③ With the movement, I'll add resistance to your hip joint.
  その動きに合わせて，股関節に抵抗を加えます。
- ④ This therapy will stimulate your adductor muscle.
  このセラピーは，内転筋を刺激し促進します。

3-3. Chronic Obstructive Pulmonary Disease (COPD)　慢性閉塞性呼吸器疾患

A. Abdominal breathing training　腹式呼吸練習

- ① Lie on your back and relax.
  仰向けに横になってリラックスしてください。
- ② I'll put a round cushion under your knees.
  膝の下に丸いクッションを置きますね。
- ③ Place one of your hands on the abdomen, and the other hand on the chest.
  片方の手をお腹に置き，もう一方の手を胸に置いてください。
- ④ Before exhaling, breathe in twice or three times.
  息を吐く前に，2回か3回息を吸っておきます。
- ⑤ Then, breathe in from the nasal cavity as you distend your stomach.
  それから，お腹をふくらませながら鼻から息を吸ってください。
- ⑥ Hold your breath for one second or two when you breathe much air.
  いっぱい息を吸ったら1～2秒ほど息を止めてください。
- ⑦ Breathe out slowly with your mouth pursed.
  口をすぼめてゆっくりと息を吐いてください。

Part 4 **Useful Expressions for Rehabilitation** リハビリテーションに役立つ英語表現

- ⑧ Make sure that you are practising the abdominal breathing by moving your hand up and down on the stomach along with the breathing.

  手をお腹に置いて，呼吸とともにお腹の手が上がったり下がったりすることで腹式呼吸を確かめます。

B. Panic control in the sitting position 座位でのパニックコントロール

- ① You are likely to panic when you become unable to breathe.

  呼吸ができなくなるとパニックになりやすいです。

- ② Before you are in dead panic, you need to control it.

  完全にパニックになる前に，コントロールすることが必要です。

- ③ When you are extremely short of breath, sit on the chair backward and hold its backrest.

  ひどく呼吸困難になったら，椅子に後ろ向きに座り，背もたれをつかみます。

- ④ Bend your upper body forward and breathe slowly.

  上半身を前方に曲げ，ゆっくり息をします。

- ⑤ So, you will calm down.

  すると落ち着くでしょう。

3-4. Peripheral Nerve Injury　末梢神経損傷

A. In the early stage　初期の段階で

- ① You bruised the upper arm when you slipped over a banana peel at the back door of your house, didn't you?

  お宅の裏口でバナナの皮にすべって腕を打撲されたのですね？

- ② If the nerves in the forearm have been injured, your hand may be bent at the wrist and to make matters worse, your fingers may not be bent.

  もし前腕の神経が損傷を受けていると，手が手首の位置で曲がり，さらに悪いことには，指は曲がらなくなります。

- ☐ ③ Fortunately, there was no apparent injury in the peripheral nerves on examination, but the radial nerves are stretched a little.

  幸い，検査では末梢神経に明らかな損傷はみられませんでしたが，橈骨神経が少し伸びています。

- ☐ ④ So, I'll perform the range of motion exercise on your hand to keep the thumb opposable to the other fingers.

  ですから，あなたの手の可動域運動を行い，親指が他の指と向かい合うようにします。

- ☐ ⑤ Warming your arm is also effective. I will bring a hot pack apparatus later.

  腕を温めるのも効果的です。あとでホットパックをお持ちします。

B. ROM (range of motion) exercise of the upper extremity
上肢可動域訓練

- ☐ ① Your body seems to be stiff while you rested quietly in bed.

  安静にしていた間に身体が硬くなったようです。

- ☐ ② Let me help you to exercise the the range of motion of your upper arm to prevent contracture.

  拘縮を防ぐために上腕の可動域の運動をします。

- ☐ ③ I'll raise your arm without bending your elbow as highly as possible.

  あなたの腕をできるだけ肘を曲げずに高く上げます。

- ☐ ④ This exercise will recover flexibility not only of the paralyzed hand but of all over the upper extremities.

  この運動は麻痺した手ばかりでなく，上肢全体の柔軟性を取り戻します。

- ☐ ⑤ Excessive extension of your hand is protected with a splint.

  添え木を当てて，手の過伸長を防いでいます。

Part 4 **Useful Expressions for Rehabilitation**　リハビリテーションに役立つ英語表現

3-5. Parkinson Disease　パーキンソン病
A. Transferring hoops to other quoits　輪投げの輪移し

- ① There are two quoits playing set here.
  ここに輪投げのセットが2セットあります。
- ② The longer pin with hoops is placed on the higher table in front of you.
  輪の付いた長い竿が目の前の高い台に置いてあります。
- ③ The other shorter pin without hoop is placed on the lower table beside you.
  輪の付いてないもう一つの短い竿がそばの低い台に置いてあります。
- ④ First, take a hoop out of the pin.
  まず，竿から一つ輪を取ります。
- ⑤ Then, turn your body to the lower table and put the hoop into the pin.
  そして，身体を低い台の方に向けてその輪を竿にかけます。
- ⑥ The motion of raising your arm to take a hoop out, turning your body, and lowering your arms to the shorter pin makes you bend and stretch the upper limbs wide.
  両腕を上げて輪を取り，身体を曲げ，短い竿まで腕を下げる動きは，上肢を広く曲げて伸ばす運動になります。
- ⑦ It also facilitates a rotation movement of your trunk.
  体幹の動きも促進します。

B. Sanding movement　サンディング

- ① Sit on the chair in front of the inclined board.
  サンディングボードの前の椅子に座ってください。
- ② Put your hand on the folded towel on the board.
  ボード上で，たたんだタオルの上に手を置いてください。
- ③ Stretch your upper limbs as high as possible, pressing the towel.
  上肢をできるだけ高く，タオルを押しながら，伸ばします。

- ④ Then, lower it to the bottom of the board.
  それから，ボードの下まで下げます。
- ⑤ The motion of rubbing with a cloth like this is called sanding.
  このように布でこする運動はサンディング運動と呼ばれます。
- ⑥ Sanding will give you a wide range of movement to your joints not to cause the bending posture.
  サンディングにより屈曲姿勢になるのを防ぐ幅広い関節の運動ができます。

3-6. Spinal Cord Injury　脊髄損傷

A. C5 complete spinal cord injury　C５完全脊髄損傷

- ① I'm afraid you experience a hard time now, but trying to move your body can be actually counterproductive more harm than good.
  今はつらい時期と思いますが，腕や手を無理に動かそうとするのは逆効果です。
- ② You should rest quietly in bed until the condition will become stable.
  安静にして，状態が落ち着くのを待ちましょう。
- ③ During the time, I'll change your position often so you don't get bedsores.
  その間，褥瘡（床ずれ）にならないように，体位を頻繁に換えます。
- ④ I also straighten up the sheet.
  シーツもきちんと整えましょう。
- ⑤ As the acute stage has passed, will you begin the range of motion exercise?
  急性期を過ぎましたから，そろそろ関節可動域の訓練を始めましょうか。
- ⑥ Raise your forearm with putting your upper arm in the spine position on the bed.

Part 4 **Useful Expressions for Rehabilitation**　リハビリテーションに役立つ英語表現

仰臥位で上腕までベッドにつけたままで，前腕を上に挙げます。

- ⑦ Bend the wrist downward as keeping the forearm raised feeling your arm very heavy.

  前腕を挙げたままで，重さを感じながら手首を下方に曲げてください。

- ⑧ I understand you are impatient to move your body freely as before, but let's try what you can do now.

  以前のように身体が自由に動かないので焦ると思いますが，できることから始めましょう。

B. Pressure elimination　除圧動作

- ① Your buttocks are sore because they have been always pressed on the wheelchair as you move anywhere.

  移動するとき常に車椅子でお尻に圧迫がかかり続けるので，褥瘡ができます。

- ② You need to do pressure elimination to prevent pressure sores.

  褥瘡を防ぐために，除圧動作の訓練を始めましょう。

- ③ First, hold the arm supports [of the wheelchair] and bend your upper body to the left and right.

  まず，アームサポートを持って，上体を左右に倒してください。

- ④ Next, let's try push-up movement training to lift the lower back high.

  次に腰を高く持ち上げるプッシュアップ動作をしてみましょう。

- ⑤ Push up your body directly above with your hands on the arm supports.

  両手をアームサポートに置いて，身体をまっすぐ上に向かって（垂直方向に）持ち上げます。

- ⑥ I'll hold your knees as the upper part of your body tends to bend forward.

  上体が前に傾かないように，私が膝を抑えておきます。

- ⑦ During your exercises, let me check if there is a space between the chair and your buttocks.

  運動の途中で,お尻の下が空いているか手を入れて確かめさせてください。

- ⑧ This exercise makes you possible to push up your body with insufficient muscle strength of your upper limbs.

  この運動は上肢筋力が不十分でも,安全に身体をプッシュアップできます。

- ⑨ Besides, we, therapists, do not hurt our lower back.

  また私たち,リハビリ士の腰も痛めません。

- ⑩ I expect you to push your body upward every thirty minutes for yourself, but please don't overdo it.

  一人でプッシュアップができるならば,30分ごとにするといいのですが,決して無理をしないでください。

C. Cervical central cord injury　中心性頚髄損傷

- ① You were involved in a traffic accident, weren't you?

  バイク事故に遭われたのですね。

- ② Severe pain and numbness of your hands cause from nerve injury in the center of the cervical cord.

  両手がひどく痛み,しびれがあるのは,頚髄の中心部分が打撃を受けて神経が傷ついているためです。

- ③ The upper part of the body is occupied with the cervical nerves.

  頚髄の神経が,上半身を支配していますから。

- ④ Fortunately, your neck is neither fractured nor injured.

  幸いにも首に骨折も傷もありません。

- ⑤ As the inside of the spine remains broad enough, the spinal cord, the very fragile nervous tissue, is not pressed.

  背骨の中は十分広いままなので,とても脆弱な神経組織である脊

髄が圧迫されていません。

☐ ⑥ Today, let's start a simple exercise of grasping a soft ball.
今日は，柔らかいボールを握る単純な練習から始めます。

☐ ⑦ Please hold the balls in your hands facing each other, and grasp them as tightly as possible.
ボールを握った手を向かい合せにして，できるかぎり強く握ってください。

☐ ⑧ You will get strong grip strength gradually as you exercise over and over again every day.
毎日，何度も練習しているうちに，力が強くなります。

☐ ⑨ I'm sure you are young enough to recover spontaneously before long.
お若いので，きっとこれから自然によくなっていきますよ。

☐ ⑩ But I believe continuous exercise patiently is most important.
でも，根気よく練習を続けることがいちばん大切だと思います。

3-7. Rheumatoid Arthritis　関節リウマチ

A. Active movement of finger joints　手指関節の自動運動

☐ ① Main treatment for rheumatoid arthritis is targeted to a reduction of sharp pain and contracture of the joints.
関節リウマチの主な治療は，関節の鋭い痛みと拘縮の軽減を目的にしています。

☐ ② I'll give you some instructions of active movements for such symptoms.
そのような症状に対する自動運動をいくつか教えます。

☐ ③ Place the back of your hands on the table, and bend the elbows.
両手の甲を台の上に置き，肘を曲げます。

☐ ④ Raise your forearm toward yourself as the palms are.
手の平をそのままに，前腕を自分の方に向かって上げます。

- ☐ ⑤ Extend all the fingers on the table, and abduct the little finger, ring finger and middle finger in succession.
  台の上で指を伸ばしてください。そして小指,薬指(環指),中指を続けて外転させます。
- ☐ ⑥ Clench your fist, and extend all fingers.
  握りこぶしを作り,指をすべて伸ばしてください。
- ☐ ⑦ Bend your first and second finger joints.
  指の第一関節と第二関節を曲げてください。
- ☐ ⑧ With fingers extended, bend the carpal joints to the side of the thumb, and then, to the little finger.
  指を伸ばしたまま,手関節を親指側へ,次に,小指側へ曲げてください。
- ☐ ⑨ One thing to keep in mind is to stop the exercise when your affected part aches.
  一つ覚えておいてほしいことは,患部が痛んだときには運動を止めることです。
- ☐ ⑩ Moreover, you should not exercise when the joints become inflamed.
  さらに,関節が炎症を起こしたときは運動しないことです。

B. Exercise for having a good posture 作業の間に良い姿勢を保つ運動

- ☐ ① Sit [down] on the edge of the bench.
  ベンチの端に座ってください。
- ☐ ② Put your left hand on your hip.
  左手を腰に置きます。
- ☐ ③ Raising the other hand, bend your body to the left.
  もう一方の手を上げ,身体を左に曲げます。
- ☐ ④ Be careful not to bend too much.
  曲げすぎないように気をつけてください。
- ☐ ⑤ Repeat the exercise on the opposite side.

Part 4 **Useful Expressions for Rehabilitation** リハビリテーションに役立つ英語表現

反対側にも繰り返してください。
- ⑥ With this gymnastic exercise, you'll be able to keep good posture.
  この体操で，良い姿勢を保つことができます。
- ⑦ Also, you can do the same exercise with a standing position.
  また，同じ運動を立った姿勢でもできます。
- ⑧ This exercise will be especially recommended when you have to continue to sit on.
  この運動は，座り続けなければならないときに，特にお勧めします。

C. Paraffin bath　パラフィン浴

- ① When the joints are not inflamed, we recommend you paraffin bath.
  関節が炎症を起こしてなければ，パラフィン浴をお勧めします。
- ② Wash your hands well and dry.
  手をよく洗って乾かします。
- ③ Put your hands in a natural way in paraffin heated and dissolved in the equipment.
  両手を自然な形で，装置の中で温め溶解したパラフィンに入れます。
- ④ Keep your hands in it only for one or two seconds, and take them out.
  両手を1〜2秒だけ入れてから出します。
- ⑤ As you repeat these motions ten times, white thin coats are piled up as a thick gloves on your hands.
  この動きを10回繰り返すと，白く薄い膜が重なり合って，厚い手袋のようになります。
- ⑥ In the last time, put your hands in for ten minutes.
  最後に，10分間そこに両手を入れたままにします。
- ⑦ In this way, your hands will be evenly warmed without getting burned.
  このようにすると，両手がやけどすることなく均等に温まります。

3-8. Dysphagia　嚥下障害

A. Warming-up exercise before meal　食前の準備運動

☐ ① The first morsel of food sometimes leads the accidental ingestion, so let's do warm-up exercises before having a meal.
食べ始めの一口に誤嚥が起きやすいので，準備運動をしましょう。

☐ ② At first, relax with abdominal breathing.
最初に腹式呼吸をしてリラックスをします。

☐ ③ Breathe in from the nose putting your hand on your abdomen.
お腹に手を軽く当ててお腹を膨らませながら鼻から息を吸います。

☐ ④ While pulling your abdomen, breathe out from your mouth.
お腹を引っ込ませながら口から息を吐いてください。

☐ ⑤ Then, move your neck slowly back and forth, right and left, and rotate it.
次に，首をゆっくりと前後，左右に動かし，ぐるりと回しましょう。

☐ ⑥ In order to pass food easily through the throat, let's move around and inside of the mouth.
食べ物をのどに送りやすくするために，口の周囲と口の中の運動をしましょう。

☐ ⑦ Say slowly "Pa, Ra, Ka" five times.
ゆっくりと「パ・ラ・カ」と5回繰り返します。

☐ ⑧ Then, repeat them five or six times as quickly as possible.
今度はできるだけ早く5，6回繰り返します。

☐ ⑨ Now, take a deep breath.
深呼吸をしましょう。

B. Before and during a meal　食前・食事中

☐ ① If food sticks your throat, you may suffocate, or if food goes into the trachea by mistake, you will be in danger of pneumonia.
食べ物がのどに詰まると窒息し，誤って気管に入ると肺炎を起こ

Part 4 **Useful Expressions for Rehabilitation**　リハビリテーションに役立つ英語表現

してとても危険です。

- ② Let me raise your bed to an angle of 30 degrees for avoiding an accidental ingestion.
  誤嚥を防ぐために，ベッドを30度に上げます。
- ③ I'll also raise your pillow, so your head will be lifted a little.
  枕を高くするので，頭が少し前向きになります。
- ④ I'll sit on your unaffected side in order to have you concentrate on your meal.
  食事に集中してもらうために，麻痺していない側で食事介助します。
- ⑤ To prevent choking food in your throat, I'll turn your neck sideways.
  食べ物がのどにひっかからないように，首を回します（横向き嚥下）。
- ⑥ I know you are thirsty, but swallowing water or juice is very difficult for you.
  のどが渇いているでしょうけれど，水やジュースを飲み下すのは難しいのです。
- ⑦ Instead, let's eat cold jelly every bite.
  代わりに，冷えたゼリーを一口ずつ食べましょう。
- ⑧ To slide down your throat easily, vegetables are thickened with starch.
  喉を通りやすいように，野菜にもとろみをつけています。
- ⑨ I'm glad you could eat all.
  全部食べられてよかったですね。
- ⑩ Now, let me clean your mouth. Oral hygiene is very important for health not only of your mouth but also other organs.
  口の中をきれいにしておきましょう。口腔衛生は口だけでなく，他の器官の健康にも重要です。

日本語索引

あ

アームスリング	32
アカラシア	80
アキレス腱	141
――滑液包炎	55
――断裂	59
――反射	150
悪性の	49
あくび	53
あぐら座位	2
握力	8
顎	114
顎の先	114
顎髭	123
あざ	76
アザラシ肢症	103
足；脚	141
足首〔の〕	141
アシドーシス	44
足取り	5
足の裏	141
足の甲	141
足踏み反射	152
足ゆび(指；趾)	141
足指義足	28
アスピリン	20
亜脱臼	57
頭	114
圧痛	52
圧迫骨折	54
圧迫包帯	34
アップアンドゴーテスト	9
アテトーゼ	66
アテトーゼ様運動	60
アデノイド肥大	48
アデノシンデアミナーゼ欠損症	101
アテローム〔性動脈〕硬化〔症〕	62
アトピー性湿疹	75
アトピー性皮膚炎	75
アドレナリン	152
アヒル歩行	60
アブミ(鐙)骨	115
アミノ酸	152
アミロイドーシス	92
アメーバ〔の〕	111
歩み	5
アルカローシス	44
歩き方	5
アルコール依存〔症〕	44, 104
アルコール中毒リハプログラム	20
アルツハイマー型認知症	105
アルツハイマー病	64
アルドステロン症	92
アレルギー〔性〕〔の〕	44
暗順応	147
暗点	122

い

胃〔の〕	134
胃炎	81
胃潰瘍	81
胃下垂	81
胃がん	81
閾値	16
胃憩室	81
井桁組み	23
椅座位	2
いざり這い	5
胃酸過多	81
胃酸減少	81
意識混濁	45
意識障害	47
意志疎通	41
萎縮〔症〕	44
異常姿勢	2
移乗動作	5
移植〔術〕	19
異食〔症〕	107
胃食道逆流性疾患	81
移植片	19
異所性ACTH症候群	92
異所性骨化	58
異所性精巣(睾丸)	102
異性愛	105
胃切除後症候群	82
依存〔症〕	46
いちご状舌	52
一次性の	50
胃腸炎	81
胃腸症	81
一回換気量	10
一過性の	52
一過性脳虚血発作	66
一歩	5
遺伝性運動失調〔症〕	102
遺伝性の	48
遺伝性光ミオクローヌス	102
移動動作	5
いびき〔をかく〕	51
いびき音	51
異物	47
いぼ	77
医療安全管理	42
医療過誤	41
医療過失	41
医療社会事業	37
医療(医薬)情報担当者	41
医療ソーシャルワーカー	36
医療面接	17
イレウス	82
院外作業療法	21
陰核	135
陰茎〔の〕	135
咽喉	131
咽喉炎	51
インスリン	153

咽頭〔の〕	131	運動障害	59, 60	円板状半月	56
咽頭炎	51, 74	運動処方	18		
咽頭がん	83	運動神経	127	**お**	
咽頭結膜熱	110	運動神経根	129	横臥位	2
咽頭反射	151	運動性言語中枢	119	横隔膜〔の〕	128
院内感染	110	運動負荷心電図検査	7	横支靱帯	137
陰嚢〔の〕	135			黄色ブドウ球菌	111
インフォームド・		**え**		凹足	57
コンセント	17	エイズ	90	横足根関節	143
陰部神経	133	栄養欠乏症	95	黄体形成(黄体化)	
陰部ヘルペス	87	栄養疾患	95	ホルモン	153
インフルエンザ	110	栄養失調	95	黄体刺激ホルモン	
インポテンス	87	エウスタキオ管	121	分泌異常症候群	93
		腋窩	128	黄疸	49
う		腋窩神経	139	嘔吐	52
ウィスコンシンカード		エコー	9	応答	152
分類検査	9	壊死	49	嘔吐感	49
ウイルス〔の〕	111	壊疽	48	横突起	125
ウイルス感染後疲弊		X脚	56	嘔吐反射	151, 152
症候群	68	エネルギー代謝率	8	黄斑	122
ウェゲナー肉芽腫症	90	エピネフリン	152	黄斑症	71
ウェスタン失語症統合		エボラウイルス	112	黄斑変性症	71
検査	9	エボラ出血熱	109	O脚	56
ウェルニッケ中枢(野)	119	エリテマトーデス	90	オーバートレーニング	
右胸心	103	エルゴメーター	32	症候群	55
右屈	3	遠位指(趾)節間関節	136	大振り歩行	60
烏口腕筋	138	遠位橈尺関節円板	137	悪寒	45
動き	25	円回内筋	139	置き梯子	33
う(齲)歯	82	遠隔操作用具	33	おくび	44
牛海綿状脳症	109	嚥下	148	おしっこする	52
右心症	103	円形脱毛症	74	悪心	49
右旋	4	嚥下機能	148	おたふくかぜ	109
内がえし	4	嚥下グレード	16	オッペンハイマー	
うちくるぶし	141	嚥下訓練	24	スプリント(副子)	31
内分回し	3	嚥下障害(困難)	80	おでき	75
うっ血性心不全	61	嚥下中枢	119	おとがい(頤)	114
うつ(鬱)病	105	嚥下痛	50	おとがい筋	116
腕	136	嚥下反射	152	おとがい舌筋	116
うなじ(項)	114	遠視	71	おとがい舌骨筋	116
運動	24, 25, 60	炎症〔性の〕	49	お腹	132
運動異常症	59	炎症性腸疾患	82	おねしょ	44
運動機能テスト	8	延髄	120	オペラント行動	12

おむつ	33	階段昇降	5	角状脊柱後弯	54
親知らず	123	階段昇降機	34	喀痰	51
オリーブ	121	回法〔の〕	134	拡張	46
オリーブ橋小脳萎縮症	67	外転	3	拡張型心筋症	61
おりもの	87	外転筋	138	角膜炎	71
音響外傷	72	外転神経	117	角膜乾燥症	70
音響反射	11	回内	4	角膜曲率測定	11
音叉	11	海馬〔の〕	120	角膜症	71
温熱療法	22	灰白質	120	角膜反射	150
温冷交替浴	25	灰白髄炎	68	過形成	146
か		外反	3	下後鋸筋	126
果(踝)〔の〕	141	外反膝	56	過呼吸症候群	78
カーク切断	18	外鼻孔	122	仮死	52
臥位	2	回復期リハビリテーション	35	下肢	141
外果	141			下肢静脈瘤	63
回外	4	外腹斜筋反射	150	下肢伸展挙上試験	9
回外筋	139	外閉鎖筋	133	下肢切断	18
外眼筋	116	解剖学的肢位	2	家事動作	5
壊血病	96	開放骨折	54	過食〔症〕	107
介護支援センター	39	潰瘍	52	下垂足	56
介護福祉士	35	潰瘍性大腸炎	80	下垂体	120
介護保険施設	39	解離性障害	105	下垂体機能亢進症	93
介護老人保健施設	39	外肋間筋	128	下垂体機能低下症	93
〔情報〕開示	41	下咽頭収縮筋	116	ガス交換	148
外耳	121	過栄養	95	かぜ	45
外耳炎	73	家屋−樹木−人物画法テスト	12	下制	3
外耳孔	114			下双子筋	144
外傷後頚部症候群	55	下顎〔骨〕〔の〕	114	家族性大腸ポリポーシス	102
外傷性脳損傷	66	下顎反射	150	家族性の	47
介助犬	33	化学療法	21	家族歴	17
回旋	4	踵	141	肩	136
疥癬	76	踵歩き	59	片足立ち	5
外旋	4	踵バンパー	32	片足立ちテスト	8
回旋筋	126	かがみ肢位	2	片足跳び	5
〔肩〕回旋筋腱板	137	過換気症候群	78	下腿義足	28
咳嗽反射	150	果義肢	26	下腿三頭筋	144
外側広筋	144	果義足	28	下腿三頭筋反射	150
外腹斜筋	132	蝸牛	121	下腿切断	18
外側大腿皮神経	145	蝸牛神経	117	肩関節	137
外側直筋	116	顎関節症	57	肩関節周囲炎	57
外側翼突筋	116	角質	123	肩義手	27
		学習障害	106	肩こり	59

肩装具	30	感覚統合療法	22	乾癬	76
肩継手	28	眼窩上神経	117	汗腺	124
片膝立ち	5	肝〔臓〕がん	82	乾癬性関節炎	56
可聴閾値；可聴範囲	147	換気性作業閾値	10	肝臓〔の〕	134
滑液包炎	56	眼球	122	環椎	114
脚気	94	眼球運動	147	眼底検査	10
滑車神経	117	眼球運動測定異常	11	眼ディスメトリア	11
褐色細胞腫	93	眼球共同運動	147	眼動脈	118
活動電位	7	眼球正位	147	冠〔状〕動脈〔性心〕疾患	61
滑脳症	103	眼球突出	70	肝斑	74
合併症	45	眼筋	116	乾皮症	77
可動域；可動性	60	ガングリオン	58	肝不全	81
角結膜炎	71	間欠性の	49	感冒	45
痂皮	74	間欠性跛行	5, 60	汗疱状白癬	76
過敏膀胱	85	肝血流量	149	感冒薬	20
下腹部痛	82	眼瞼下垂	70	陥没骨折	54
花粉症	74	肝硬変	80	顔面筋反射	150
カポジ肉腫	76	寛骨	132	顔面紅潮	47
痒み	49	寛骨臼	132	顔面神経	117
殻構造義肢	26	肝細胞がん	81	緘黙症	106
カリウム枯渇	95	カンジダ	111	眼輪筋	116
仮義肢	26	カンジダ症	109	眼輪筋反射	151
仮義手	27	癌腫	146		
仮義足	28	肝腫大	81	**き**	
カルチノイド	146	肝障害	81	既往歴	17
カルチノイド症候群	92	感情障害	104	記憶障害	47
カルメット-ゲラン菌(BCG)ワクチン	22	冠状動脈	129	気管〔の〕	131
加齢黄斑変性症	71	感情鈍麻	64	気管支〔の〕	131
革細工	23	感情不一性致精神病	106	気管支炎	78
革装具	29	眼精疲労	70	気管支拡張症	78
がん	146	関節運動学的アプローチ	17	気管支拡張薬	20
〔脈〕管	130	関節炎	56	気管支原性〔肺〕がん	78
眼圧測定〔法〕	11	関節可動域訓練	24	気管軟骨	131
簡易上肢機能テスト	9	関節可動域テスト	8	気管分岐部	131
簡易知能検査	12	関節形成(置換)術	18	危機管理	41
肝炎	81	関節拘縮	56	利き手交換	23
眼窩〔の〕	115	関節固定術	18	気胸	79
寛解	18, 51	関節痛	56	奇形症候群	103
感覚異常	68	関節変形	56	起座呼吸	78
感覚性言語中枢	119	関節リウマチ	57	義肢装具訓練	24
感覚中枢	119	関節離断〔術〕	18, 56	義肢・装具士	35
		感染〔性の〕	49	義肢・装具療法	21

気腫	78	臼歯	123	強直性脊椎炎	55
基準	14	吸収不良症候群	95	胸椎装具	31
寄生生物;寄生虫	111	球状足関節	141	共同〔性〕注視	147
偽性低アルドステロン症	94	丘疹	76	強迫性障害	106
偽性副甲状腺機能低下症	94	嗅神経	117	強皮症	76
気絶	47	急性期リハビリテーション	35	恐怖〔症〕	107
基礎血圧	7	急性ストレス障害	104	強膜〔の〕	122
基礎代謝率	8	急性の	44	胸膜炎	78
ぎっくり腰	55	吸息	148	胸膜中皮腫	78
気道	131	吸着式ソケット	26	胸膜斑(プラーク)	50
亀頭包皮炎	87	吸着式大腿義足	29	共有性精神病性障害	108
キヌタ(砧)骨	115	救命処置	17	胸肋関節	128
機能回復訓練事業	37	橋	121	棘下筋	126
機能〔回復〕訓練	24	胸〔部〕	128	棘上筋	139
機能障害	47	教育のリハビリテーション	35	虚血性心疾患	62
機能の作業療法	22	仰臥位	2	虚血性脳血管障害	65
機能の残気量	10	胸郭	128	挙睾筋反射	150
機能の肢位	2	胸管	129	距骨〔の〕	143
機能の自立度評価法	8	狂牛病	109	距骨下関節	143
機能の電気刺激〔法〕	21	頬筋	115	距骨傾斜	143
機能不全	47	挙上	3
亀背	54	胸腔	128	距踵舟関節	143
希発月経	88	狂犬病	110	巨人症	93
ギプス	34	頬骨	115	距腿関節	143
ギプス副子(シーネ)	34	胸骨〔の〕	128	巨大結腸症	82
気分障害	106	頬骨神経	117	巨大脳髄腫	103
気分変調性障害	105	胸最長筋	128	起立	5
木彫り	23	胸鎖関節	128	起立性低血圧〔症〕	63
基本の救命処置	17	狭窄性腱鞘炎	59	偽リンパ腫	146
基本の肢位	2	強擦法	25	キルティング	23
基本日常生活動作	4	胸鎖乳突筋	129	亀裂骨折	54
虐待	44	胸神経	129	近位指節間関節	137
脚長差	5	狭心症	61	筋萎縮〔症〕	58
逆ナックルベンダー	32	胸水	47	筋萎縮性側索硬化症	68
ギャッジ(ギャッチ)ベッド	33	矯正器具	34	近位(上)橈尺関節	137
キャッチ22症候群	101	胸腺	129	筋緊張性ジストロフィー	58
嗅覚過敏	74	胸腺過形成	100	近見反射	151
嗅覚障害;嗅覚消失	73	蟯虫症	109	筋硬直	58
嗅覚鈍麻	73	協調性訓練	23	筋再教育訓練	23
嗅球	123	協調性テスト	7	近視	71
救急処置室	38	胸腸肋筋	126	筋弛緩訓練	23
球菌〔の〕	111	〔関節〕強直〔症〕	55	筋ジストロフィー	58

項目	ページ
筋層	134
金属枠装具	29
緊張性昏迷	104
筋電義手	27
筋電図	7
筋電図検査〔法〕	8
筋肉固定術	19
筋肉増強訓練	23
筋無力〔症〕症候群	58
筋無力症	58
筋力低下	58

く

項目	ページ
空間視力	152
空腸〔の〕	138
くしゃみ	53
口すぼめ呼吸	26
口尖らし反射	156
口髭	128
靴型装具	33
屈曲	3, 4
屈筋反射	155
クッシング病	94
クッシング様顔貌	97
屈折検査	12
靴べら式装具	33
くも膜	123
くも膜下腔	125
くも膜下出血	68
グラスゴー昏睡尺度	17
クラッチ	34
クラプの匍匐運動	26
クラミジア	114
クラミジア肺炎	81
クリティカルパス	43
クループ	80
グループホーム	41
グループ訓練	26
グルテン性腸症	82
踝〔の〕	141
くる病	98
車椅子	35

項目	ページ
車椅子動作	5
クレイグ・ハンディキャップ評価・報告法	14
グレーブズ病	95
クレンザック継手	31
クロイツフェルト－ヤコブ病	69
訓練	26

け

項目	ページ
ケアハウス	39
ケアマネジメント	37
ケアマネジャー	35
頚〔部〕〔の〕	114
頚棘筋	126
頚肩腕症候群	56
脛骨〔の〕	143
脛骨神経	145
頚最長筋	116
軽擦法	25
傾斜台	34
痙縮	51
芸術療法	22
茎状突起	137
頚静脈	118
頚神経	117
頚〔部脊〕髄	120
頚髄損傷	65
形成異常〔症〕	47
頚長筋	116
頚腸肋筋	126
頚椎	114
頚椎装具	31
痙動	52
頚動脈	118
頚動脈結節	114
頚板状筋	126
経皮的電気刺激〔法〕	21
軽費老人ホーム	39
頚部脊中管狭窄症	54
鶏歩	60
傾眠	51

項目	ページ
痙攣	45
ケースマネジメント	37
ケースワーカー	35
ケースワーク	37
劇症性の	47
激痛	50
下剤	20
化粧室	33
血圧	7
血圧測定	9
血液脳関門	119
〔肺〕結核	79
血管炎	62
血管炎症候群	63
血管拡張(弛緩)薬	20
血管雑音	63
血管迷走神経症候群	69
月経異常	87
月経困難症	87
月経前緊張症(症候群)	88
結合部	26
血色素尿症	97
血漿	146
血小板	146
血小板血症	100
血小板減少症	100
血清	146
血精液症	87
血清反応陰性脊椎炎	90
結節性甲状腺腫	93
血栓	52
血栓性静脈炎	63
血栓溶解薬	20
欠損〔症〕	46
血痰	51
結腸	134
結腸がん	80
血尿	84
げっぷ	44
欠乏〔症〕	46
結膜炎	70
結膜反射	150

血友病	97	更衣動作	4	高コレステロール血症	94
ケトアシドーシス	93	抗うつ薬	19	後根神経節	127
解毒薬	19	高栄養療法	21	虹彩	122
解熱薬	20	抗炎症薬	19	高脂血症	94
下痢	80	構音障害	52, 65	高次脳機能障害	65
下痢止め	19	構音不能〔症〕	64	後十字靭帯	142
ケルニッヒ徴候	16	口蓋〔の〕	123	後縦靭帯	142
腱移行術；腱移植術	19	〔軟〕口蓋音	52	後縦靭帯骨化症	58
牽引療法	22	口蓋骨	115	拘縮	45, 58
腱炎	59	口蓋心顔面症候群	103	甲状腺	114
幻覚	105	口蓋垂	123	甲状腺炎	94
検眼	10	口蓋扁桃	123	甲状腺機能亢進症	93
肩甲下筋	139	口蓋裂	102	甲状腺機能低下症	93
肩甲挙筋	139	光覚	147	甲状腺結節	93
肩甲骨	128	口角下制筋	115	甲状腺刺激ホルモン	153
肩甲上腕関節	136	口角挙筋	116	——受容体異常症	94
健康診断	7	高額療養費支給制度	37	——放出ホルモン	153
言語障害	46, 66	硬化症	68	甲状腺腫瘍	94
言語中枢	119	高カリウム血症	94	甲状腺ホルモン不応症	94
言語聴覚士	36	高カルシウム血症	94	口唇ヘルペス	109
腱索	130	睾丸〔の〕	135	向精神薬	20
犬歯	123	交感神経幹	121	硬性装具	29
幻視	105	抗凝固薬	19	厚生年金制度	37
幻肢痛	50	口峡反射	150	抗生物質	19
肩手症候群	55	咬筋	116	光線過敏症	71
腱鞘炎	59	咬筋反射	151	酵素	152
剣状突起	128	抗菌薬	19	梗塞〔症〕	49
倦怠感	47	口腔	123	後退	4
原虫	111	口腔アフタ	83	抗体	152
幻聴	72, 105	後傾位	2	高体温症	48
見当識障害	46, 65	後脛骨筋	144	叩打法	25
減捻装具	32	硬結	51	好中球減少症	99
原発性の	50	高血圧〔症〕	63	硬直	51
腱反射	152	抗血栓薬	19	光痛〔症〕	71
肩峰	136	抗原	152	交通動脈	118
健忘〔症〕	104	抗高脂血症治療薬	19	口蹄病	109
肩峰下〔滑液〕包	137	交互式三点歩行	59	後天性の	44
		交互対光反応試験	11	後天性免疫不全症候群	90
こ		後骨間神経	139	喉頭〔の〕	131
降圧薬	19	交互ひきずり歩行	60	喉頭炎	73
抗アレルギー薬	19	交互歩行器	33	喉頭蓋	131
行為障害	104	交互歩行装具	30	喉頭蓋軟骨	131

喉頭がん	73	股関節	132	骨肉腫	55
後頭筋	116	股関節伸展筋歩行	60	骨盤〔の〕	132
喉頭口	131	股関節部	125	骨盤帯付き長下肢装具	30
後頭骨	115	〔努力〕呼気肺活量	10	骨半規管	121
行動性無視検査	7	呼吸〔の〕	24, 149	固定	59
後頭前頭筋	116	呼吸音	149	拳	136
喉頭反射	151	呼吸機能	149	小振り歩行	60
行動評価	13	呼吸筋	128	鼓膜	121
喉頭ポリープ	73	呼吸訓練	23	鼓膜炎	72
喉頭隆起	120	呼吸困難	78	こめかみ〔の〕	114
高度救命処置	17	呼吸商	149	コモードチェア	33
口内炎	82	呼吸中枢	119	コレステロール	152
高尿酸血症	94	呼吸抵抗	10	コレラ	109
高熱	47	呼吸不全	79	混合性結合組織病	90
更年期障害(症候群)	87	呼吸麻痺	79	昏睡	45
広背筋	126	呼吸リハビリテーション	35	コンピュータ断層撮影診断〔法〕	7
紅斑	75	刻印打ち	23	昏迷	52
後半月大腿靭帯	142	黒色腫	76	混乱	45
紅斑性狼瘡	90	国民健康保険	37		
後鼻孔	122	腰	125	**さ**	
紅皮症	76	帯下	87		
抗ヒスタミン薬	19	固執傾向	50	座位	2
抗不安薬	19	五十肩	57	細気管支〔の〕	131
後方挙上	3, 4	固縮	45, 51	細菌〔の〕	111
硬膜	120	股装具	30	細菌性食中毒	109
硬膜下血腫	66	呼息	148	細静脈	130
硬膜下腔	121	呼息筋	128	臍静脈	133
硬膜下出血	66	骨炎	55	最大換気(吸気)量	10
肛門〔の〕	134	骨化〔症〕	58	在宅ケア	37
肛門括約筋	132	骨格構造義肢	26	在宅〔福祉〕サービス	37
肛門挙筋	133	骨格構造義足	28	在宅リハビリテーション	37
抗リウマチ薬	20	骨形成不全症	55	臍動脈	133
抗利尿ホルモン	153	骨系統疾患	55	催吐反射	151
――分泌異常症候群	93	骨髄異形成症候群	99	サイトメガロウイルス	112
口輪筋	116	骨髄腫	99	採尿器	34
抗リン脂質抗体症候群	90	骨髄線維症	99	再評価	15
高齢者生活福祉センター	39	骨髄増殖疾患群	99	座位保持装具	29
〔脊柱〕後弯〔症〕	54	骨折	54	催眠薬	20
氷マッサージ	25	骨接合術	19	サイム義足	29
語音聴取閾値	11	骨粗鬆症	55	サイム切断	18
語音聴力検査	11	骨〔伝〕導	11	サヴァン症候群	107
語音明瞭度〔検査〕	11	骨軟化症	55	作業耐容性	9

作業用義手	27	耳介	121	四肢麻痺	68
作業療法	21	紫外線療法	22	歯周病	83
作業療法士	35	視角	148	思春期早発症	93
錯語〔症〕	106	視覚	148	視床〔の〕	121
左屈	3	痔核	81	視床下部〔の〕	120
鎖肛症	101	視覚失調	71	視床手	52
鎖骨〔の〕	136	視覚障害者更生施設	40	自助介助運動	24
坐骨〔の〕	132	視覚認知検査	11	自助具	33
鎖骨下筋	139	視覚フィードバック	148	視診	17
鎖骨下動脈(静脈)	129	耳下腺炎	73	指伸筋	138
坐骨神経	133	弛緩	51	視神経	117
坐骨神経痛	68	耳管	121	視神経円板	122
差し込み用ソケット	26	耳管狭窄(閉塞)症	73	歯髄炎	83
匙状爪	51	色覚	147	指数	15
挫傷	45	色覚異常	70	ジスキネジア	59
嗄声	48	磁気共鳴画像〔法〕	8	ジストニー	58
左旋	4	磁気共鳴血管造影〔法〕	8	ジストニー運動	60
痤瘡	74	色弱	70	ジストロフィー	47
雑音	49	色素脱失	75	姿勢	2
サッチ足部	28	色素沈着	76	姿勢訓練	24
サルコイドーシス	90	子宮〔の〕	135	〔手の〕指節骨	137
猿手	69	子宮筋腫	88	〔足の〕趾節骨	142
サルモネラ菌	111	子宮頚	135	歯槽	114
三角筋	138	子宮頚がん	87	歯槽炎	82
三角筋反射	150	糸球体〔の〕	135	歯槽弓	114
三角骨	137	糸球体腎炎	84	歯槽突起	114
三脚杖	32	子宮内膜症	87	持続的多動運動療法	22
残気量	10	子宮肉腫	88	舌〔の〕	123
三叉神経	117	子宮破裂	88	耳朶	121
三肢麻痺	69	死腔	148	肢体不自由児施設	39
酸素解離曲線	149	軸椎	114	肢体不自由者(児)	36
酸素消費〔量〕	149	耳硬化症	73	耳痛	72
酸素摂取〔量〕	149	視〔神経〕交叉	121	膝窩	141
酸素摂取(吸収)量	10	篩骨	114	膝蓋腱	142
残存機能	15	篩骨迷路	114	膝蓋腱反射	151
残聴	73	自己免疫性の	44	膝蓋骨〔の〕	142
三点〔動作〕歩行	59	しこり	49	膝蓋大腿関節	142
三点歩行	60	示指伸筋	138	膝窩筋	144
残尿感	86	脂質異常症	94	膝窩静脈;膝窩動脈	145
		脂質尿症	84	膝窩リンパ節	145
し		支持的作業療法	21	疾患	46
ジェネリック医薬品	20	支持部	26	失禁	49

失血	45	視野	147	縦靱帯	142
失見当識	46	社会生活技能訓練	24	重度身体障害者保護作業所	40
失語〔症〕	64	社会的入院	37	十二指腸〔の〕	134
失行〔症〕	64	社会福祉士	36	十二指腸炎	80
失構語〔症〕	64	社会リハビリテーション	35	十二指腸潰瘍	80
膝座位	2	社会歴	17	十二指腸がん	80
失算症	64	弱視	70	揉捏法	25
失書〔症〕	64	尺側手根屈筋(伸筋)	138	18トリソミー症候群	102
失神	47, 52	尺側内転	3	終末期医療	35
湿疹	75	ジャクソン型発作	59	羞明	71
失声〔症〕	64	尺度	15	手関節	137
失調〔症〕	49, 58, 65	灼熱感	45	手関節背屈装具	31
失読〔症〕	64	灼熱痛	50, 66	粥状硬化〔症〕	62
失認〔症〕	64	若年〔性〕の	49	縮瞳	147
失文法〔症〕	64	斜頚	55	手根〔の〕	136
七宝焼き	23	視野欠損	72	手根管	139
失明	70	瀉下薬	20	手根間関節	137
質問票	15	視野検査	11	手根管症候群	66
失立発作	44	斜視〔の〕	70, 71	手根中央関節	137
自転車エルゴメーター	32	視野障害	46	手根中手関節	136
〔外〕耳道	121	遮断	46	手根中手義手	27
自動運動	25	尺屈	3, 4	授産所(施設)	40
児童相談所	39	しゃっくり	48	種子骨	137, 143
自動体外式除細動器	20	尺骨〔の〕	137	手術歴	17
児童福祉施設	39	尺骨静脈	140	手掌〔の〕	136
自動歩行	6	尺骨神経	139	受精；授精	89
歯肉〔の〕	123	尺骨神経管症候群	57	主訴	45
歯肉炎	82	尺骨動脈	140	主題統覚検査	13
歯肉出血	82	ジャンパー膝	56	腫脹	47, 146
視能訓練士	35	縦隔腫瘍	78	出血	48
紫斑〔病〕	76, 100	充血	48	出血熱	109
しびれ〔感〕	50	重鎖病	97	出産	88
しびん	34	13トリソミー症候群	103	出生体重	88
ジフテリア	109	十字靱帯	142	手動点字タイプライター	32
自閉症	104	収縮	59	手動の	136
嗜癖	44	重症急性呼吸器症候群	79	手部義手	27
四辺形ソケット	26	重症筋無力症	58	腫瘍	48, 146
脂肪肝	81	舟状骨	137, 142	腫瘤	146
脂肪酸	152	重症心身障害者(児)	36	純音聴力検査	11
脂肪症	94	重症遅進児施設	38	〔視性〕瞬目反射	150, 151
しみ	74	重心	5	上咽頭炎	73
指紋	136	終神経	117	上咽頭収縮筋	116

上咽頭神経	117	焦点〔運動〕発作	66	食道逆流	81
小円筋	139	情動障害	104	食道静脈瘤	63
障害	46, 48	情動不安定	47	食欲不振	44, 104
消化管	134	小児性愛	106	食欲抑制薬	1
上顎〔骨〕〔の〕	114	小児〔性〕の	49	所方	47
上顎がん	83	小脳〔の〕	120	処方	18
消化性潰瘍	82	上皮小体機能亢進症	93	徐脈	61
消化不良	82	上皮小体機能低下症	93	シリコン製義手	27
消化薬	20	小胞炎	74	シリコン製内ソケット	26
小胸筋	128	漿膜〔の〕	134	自律訓練法	24
小頬骨筋	117	静脈〔の〕	129	自律神経失調症	69
笑筋	116	静脈炎	63	止痢薬	19
掌屈	4	静脈瘤	63	視力	148
上後鋸筋	126	睫毛	122	視力回復運動	11
猩紅熱	110	〔栄養性〕消耗症	95	視力矯正検査	11
踵骨〔の〕	141	常用義足	28	視力検査〔表〕	11
踵骨腱	141	小腰筋	126	視力障害〔低下〕	72
踵骨反射	150	小菱形筋	126	シレジアバンド	32
証拠に基づいた医療	17	小菱形骨	137	耳漏	72
上肢	136	上腕〔の〕	136	痔瘻	80
小指(趾)外転筋	138, 143	上腕義手	27	白なまず	77
小指球筋	139	上腕筋	138	心アミロイドーシス	61
小視症	106	上腕骨〔の〕	137	腎アミロイドーシス	85
小指伸筋	138	上腕骨骨折	54	人為的エラー	41
上肢切断	18	上腕三頭筋	139	腎盂腎炎	85
硝子体	122	上腕三頭筋反射	152	腎炎	84
小指(趾)対立筋	139, 144	上腕静脈	140	人格障害	106
常時二点支持歩行	59	上腕切断	18	新型コロナウイルス感染症	109
症状	52	上腕動脈	140	心窩部	128
小静脈	130	上腕二頭筋	138	腎〔臓〕がん	85
小人症	92	初期評価	14	心気症	105
上双子筋	144	職業訓練	24	深吸気量	10
踵足	57	職業リハビリテーション	35	腎虚血	86
掌側外転	3	職業病	17	真菌	111
掌側骨間筋	139	職業前作業療法	22	心筋〔の〕	130
掌側指動脈	140	食事性カルシウム欠乏症	94	心筋梗塞〔症〕	62
掌側内転	3	食事動作	4	心筋症	61
踵足歩行	59	触診	18	神経因性膀胱炎	85
小腸	134	じょく(褥)瘡〔性潰瘍〕	75	神経原性疼痛	50
小殿筋	144	食道〔の〕	134	神経膠腫	67
小転子	142	食道炎	81	神経症	106
上殿神経	145	食道がん	80		

神経性食思不振		身体化障害	108	膵臓〔の〕	134
（無食欲）症	104	身体醜形障害	104	錐体外路〔運動〕系	120
神経性大食症	104	身体障害者（児）	36	錐体交叉	121
神経生理学的アプローチ	17	身体障害者手帳	37	錐体突起	115
神経線維腫〔症〕	67, 103	身体障害者福祉法	37	錐体路	121
神経痛	67	身体障害の	46	錐体路障害	68
神経伝導速度	8	身体的依存	46	垂直吊り下げ試験	9
神経発達学的治療	17	身体表現性障害	108	水痘	111
腎硬化症	85	診断	17	水頭症	102
人工関節置換術	18	身長	8	水平外転	3
人工骨頭置換術	18	陣痛	89	水平屈曲	3, 4
人工授精	89	心停止	61	水平伸展	3
進行性骨化性線維		心的外傷後ストレス障害	107	水平内転	3
異形成症	102	伸展	3	水疱	74
腎梗塞	86	心電図検査〔法〕	7	水疱性角膜症	71
心耳	130	腎動脈	133	髄膜〔の〕	121
深指屈筋	138	心内膜	130	髄膜炎	65
心室〔の〕	130	心内膜炎	61	髄膜腫	65
心室中隔欠損〔症〕	62	腎尿細管性アシドーシス	86	睡眠	148
滲出	47	腎尿細管不全	86	睡眠開始	148
腎症	84	塵肺症	79	睡眠構造	148
尋常性魚鱗癬	76	心肺蘇生法	21	睡眠効率	148
尋常性白斑	77	心拍数	8	睡眠時驚愕症	106
深掌動脈弓	140	真皮〔の〕	123	睡眠時無呼吸症候群	79
心身症	107	深腓骨神経	145	睡眠周期	148
心身障害者（児）	36	深部温熱療法	22	睡眠障害	46, 108
心身リラクゼーション療法	22	心不全	61	睡眠段階	148
腎性骨ジストロフィー		腎不全	86	睡眠発作	67
（異栄養症）	96	心房〔の〕	130	睡眠薬	20
新生児〔性の〕	49, 89	心房中隔欠損〔症〕	62	頭蓋	115
真性赤血球増加症	100	蕁麻疹	77	頭蓋表筋	115
新生物	146	診療評価	13	頭痛	48
腎〔結〕石	86			ストーマ	32
振戦, 震顫	66	**す**		ストライド〔長；幅〕	6
心尖	130	随意運動	25	ストレッチ運動	25
心臓〔の〕	130	〔脳脊〕髄液	147	脛	141
腎臓〔の〕	135	膵〔臓〕炎	82	スピーチオージオグラム	11
心臓腫瘍	61	膵〔臓〕がん	82	スピロメーター	10
心臓突然死	62	水腫	47	スポーツ用義足	28
心臓弁膜症	62	水晶体	122		
心臓発作	62	水腎症	84	**せ**	
心臓リハビリテーション	35	スイスロック式膝継手	33	背	125

精液	135	整腸薬	20	舌炎	82
精液瘤	88	性[的]倒錯[症]	107	石灰沈着	45
生活関連動作	4	青年の	49	舌下神経	117
生活健忘チェックリスト	12	整復[術]	19	舌がん	82
生活習慣[指導]	17	精密検査	7	赤血球	146
生活習慣病	95	声門	131	赤血球増加症	97
[日常]生活の質	15	整容動作	4	舌骨	115
生活療法	22	生理痛	87	接種	21
[輸]精管	135	生理的死腔	148	癤腫症	75
性感染症	88	咳	45	摂食障害	105
性交不能症	87	赤外線療法	21	接触皮膚炎	75
正座位	2	脊髄[の]	125, 127	癤の多発症	75
精索捻転症	88	脊髄運動ニューロン	148	切断	18
精子	135	脊髄炎	67	背骨	125
清拭	25	脊髄延髄脊髄反射	151	セリアック病	80
脆弱X症候群	102	脊髄空洞症	69	前鋸筋	129
生殖不能	89	脊髄疾患	69	仙棘筋	126
精神安定薬	20	脊髄症	67	前屈	4
精神医学的リハビリテーション	35	脊髄障害	67	前傾位	2
成人呼吸窮迫(促迫)症候群	78	脊髄神経	127	前脛骨筋	144
		脊髄神経節	127	尖圭コンジローム症	87
精神障害	46	脊髄進行性筋萎縮症	58	潜伏	50
精神遅滞	106	脊髄髄節(分節)	127	仙骨[の]	125
精神的高揚	47	脊髄性筋萎縮症	58	前骨間神経	127
精神病	107	脊髄損傷	69	仙骨神経	127
精神保健福祉士	36	脊髄反射	151	仙骨神経叢	127
精神保健福祉センター	38	脊柱[管]	125	潜在的エラー	41
		脊柱狭窄症	55	浅指屈筋	138
性腺刺激ホルモン	153	脊柱起立筋	126	前斜角筋	116
——放出ホルモン	153	脊柱・骨髄腫瘍	55	前十字靭帯	142
精巣[の]	135	脊柱すべり症	55	前縦靭帯	142
精巣腫瘍	88	脊柱変形	57	浅掌動脈弓	140
精巣上体炎	87	脊椎[の]	125	前床突起	114
臍帯	135	脊椎炎	55	染色体症候群	102
声帯[ヒダ]	131	脊椎症	55	全身倦怠感	48
声帯結節	74	脊椎造影検査	8	全身性骨疾患	55
声帯麻痺	74	脊椎分離[症]	55	尖足	56
正中神経	139	咳止め	20	喘息	78
成長	48	[説明報告]責任	41	先端巨大症	92
成長ホルモン	153	赤痢	109	仙腸装具	31
		癤	75	疝痛	45
		舌咽神経	117	前庭感覚	148

前庭姿勢反射	152	増殖	146	鼡径ヘルニア	82
前庭神経	117	装飾義肢	26	組織球増殖症	97
前庭脊髄反射	152	装飾用義手	27	側頭頭頂筋	117
前庭反射	152	痩身化	53	足根〔の〕	141
前庭水管	118	総胆管	134	足根間関節	142
先天性欠損症	102	総胆管結石症	80	足根管症候群	69
先天性股関節脱白	56	総腸骨静脈(静脈)	133	足根義足	28
先天性心疾患	102	総腓骨神経	145	足根骨	143
先天性水腎症	102	象皮病	97	足根中足義足	28
先天性の	45	躁病	106	足根中足関節	143
先天性表皮水疱症		僧帽筋	126	外がえし	3
先天性副腎皮質過形成	102	僧帽弁	130	そとくるぶし	141
先天性無痛無汗症	102	僧帽弁狭窄症	62	外分回し	3
前頭筋	116	瘙痒〔症〕	49, 76	**た**	
尖頭合指〔症〕	101	早老症	103		
前頭骨	115	ソーシャルワーカー	36	ダーメンコルセット	31
前突	4	ソーシャルワーク	37	タール様便	82
先入観	41	ソーセージ状指	51	ダイアゴナルソケット	26
全肺気量	10	足アーチ	141	体位排痰法	25
浅腓骨神経	145	側臥位	2	大円筋	139
線分二等分試験	8	側屈	3	体外受精	89
前方挙上	3, 4	足趾反射	152	体外力源義肢	26
喘鳴	53	塞栓	47	体格指数	13
洗面所	33	足底〔の〕	141	大胸筋	128
せん妄	105	足底筋	144	大頬骨筋	117
前立腺〔の〕	135	足底筋反射	151	大結節	142
前立腺炎	85	足底腱膜	144	大〔後頭〕孔	114
前立腺炎症候群	85	足底腱膜反射	150	対光反射	151
前立腺がん	85	足底接地	5	第3腓骨筋	143
前立腺結石	85	足底装具	30	胎児〔性〕〔の〕	89
前立腺症	85	足底反射	151	大視症	106
前立腺膿瘍	85	側頭〔の〕	114	代謝率	8
前立腺肥大症	85	側頭筋	116	体重	9
前立腺膀胱炎	85	側頭骨	115	体重減少	53
〔脊柱〕前弯〔症〕	55	足背動脈	145	体重測定	9
前腕	136	続発性の	51	対称性緊張性頚反射	152
前腕義手	27	側腹〔部〕	132	帯状疱疹(ヘルペス)	110
そ		側副靭帯	142	大静脈	130
		側腹痛	81	体性感覚誘発電位	9
躁うつ病	106	〔脊柱〕側弯〔症〕	55	大腿〔の〕	141
双極性障害	106	側弯症装具	31	大腿義足	28
爪上皮	136	鼡径部	132	大腿筋膜張筋	144

大腿骨	142	多系統萎縮症	67	単純骨折	54
大腿骨頚部	142	多幸症	105	単純ヘルペス	109
大腿骨頚部骨折	54	多呼吸	79	単純ヘルペスウイルス	112
大腿静脈	145	多指症	103		
大腿神経	145	打診	18	短掌筋	139
大腿切断	18	多腺性内分泌不全症	93	短小指(趾)屈筋	138, 144
大腿直筋	144	ただれ	51	男性化	93, 94
大腿動脈	145	脱臼	56	弾性線維症	75
大腿二頭筋	143	脱肛	80	胆石〔症〕	80
大腿二頭筋反射	150	脱出椎間板	54	炭疽	109
大腿方形筋	144	脱水症	46	炭疽菌	111
大腿四頭筋	144	脱腸	80	断続性ラ音	45
大腸	134	脱毛〔症〕	74	短対立スプリント(副子)	31
大腸炎	80	脱抑制	46		
大腸がん	80	脱力〔感〕	47, 53	短対立装具	30
大腸菌	111	脱力発作	66	断端痛	50
大殿筋	144	多点杖	32	短橈側手根伸筋	138
大殿筋歩行	59	多動運動	25	丹毒	109
大転子	142	他動運動	25	短内転筋	132
大動脈〔の〕	129	多動性障害	105	胆嚢	134
大動脈弓	129	多糖類	153	胆嚢炎	80
大動脈弁	129	ダニ刺症	109	胆嚢がん	81
大動脈弁逆流〔症〕	61	多尿〔症〕	85	蛋白〔質〕	153
大動脈弁閉鎖〔症〕	61	多〔発性〕囊胞腎	85	蛋白質エネルギー栄養障害	95
大動脈弁閉鎖不全〔症〕	61	多発〔性〕筋炎	59	蛋白尿	85
		多発〔性〕筋炎/皮膚筋炎	59	断端訓練	24
大動脈瘤	62	多発〔性〕血管炎	63	短腓骨筋	143
大内転筋	132	多発〔性〕硬化〔症〕	69	短母指外転筋	138
体内力源義肢	26	多発〔性〕動脈炎	63	短母指(趾)屈筋	138, 144
体内力源義手	27	卵形の	135	短母指(趾)伸筋	138, 143
大脳	120	〔男性型〕多毛	75	単麻痺	67
大脳基底核	119	多裂筋	126	断裂	59
胎盤〔の〕	135	痰	51		
大腰筋	126	単核球症	99	**ち**	
対立	4	短下肢装具	30	チアノーゼ	45
大菱形筋	126	胆管炎	80	チアミン欠乏症	96
大菱形骨	137	単光子放射断層撮影〔法〕	9	地域リハビリテーション	37
多飲	50	端座位	2	蓄膿症	74
唾液腺	123	段差解消機	33	恥骨〔の〕	132
唾液腺萎縮	83	短趾屈筋	144	恥骨筋	133
唾液腺腫瘍	83	単軸ひざ	29	智歯	123
他覚的聴力検査	11	短趾伸筋	143	腟〔の〕	135

知的障害	106
知的障害児通園施設	38
知的障害児童施設	39
知的障害者(児)	36
知能指数	15
遅発性の	52
チフス	111
恥毛	124
チャージ連合〔症候群〕	101
注意欠陥/多動性障害	104
中咽頭収縮筋	116
中隔〔の〕	130
中間広筋	144
肘筋	138
中腰位	2
注視	147
中耳	121
中耳炎	73
注射〔器〕	21
中手〔の〕	136
中手骨	137
中手指節関節	137
虫垂	134
虫垂炎	80
中枢	119
中枢神経〔系〕	117
中足〔の〕	141
中足アーチ	142
中足骨	142
中足趾節関節	142
中足骨バー	30
中殿筋	144
中殿筋歩行	60
肘頭	136
中毒	44, 50
中脳	121
中鼻甲介	115
昼盲〔症〕	70
虫様筋	139
腸〔の〕	134
腸炎	80
超音波検査〔法〕	9

聴覚	147
聴覚失認	72
聴覚消失(障害)	72
聴覚疲労	72
長下肢装具	30
蝶形骨	115
蝶形骨洞	123
腸脛靱帯	142
徴候	16
腸骨〔の〕	132
腸骨筋	132
長座位	2
長趾屈筋	144
長趾伸筋	143
長掌筋	139
聴診	17
聴神経	117
聴神経腫瘍	72
長対立スプリント(副子)	31
長対立装具	29
腸チフス	110
長橈側手根伸筋	138
腸内細菌	111
長内転筋	132
長腓骨筋	143
重複障害者(児)	36
重複歩〔長;幅〕	6
腸閉塞〔症〕	82
長母指外転筋	138
長母指(趾)屈筋	139, 144
長母指(趾)伸筋	138, 143
超早熟児	88
腸腰筋	132
聴力	147
聴力検査	11
直腸〔の〕	134
直腸がん	82
直立位	3
治療	22
治療的電気刺激〔法〕	21
治療プログラム	18
治療薬	20

治療用装具	29
鎮咳薬	20
鎮静薬	20
鎮痛薬	19

つ

椎間孔	125
椎間板	125
椎間板造影術	19
椎間板内圧	148
椎間板ヘルニア	54
椎骨〔の〕	125
椎骨動脈	118
対麻痺	68
痛覚過敏	48
通所リハビリテーション	37
——サービス	37
痛風	94
痛風結節	48
杖	32
疲れ目	70
継手〔関節〕	26
つたい歩き	6
ツチ(槌)骨	115
つま先立ち	5
爪	136

て

手〔の〕	136
手足口病	109
低栄養	52
低温療法	22
低カリウム血症	95
低カルシウム血症	94
定期健診	7
底屈	4
低血圧〔症〕	63
低血糖症	48
抵抗運動	25
低周波療法	22
低身長	92
底側骨間筋	144

低体温症	48			頭板状筋	126
低蛋白血症	95	**と**		頭皮	124
ティネル徴候	16	トイレ	33	頭部ふらふら感	49
適応障害	104	トイレ動作	5	動脈〔の〕	129
手義手	27	同一性障害	105	動脈炎	62
笛声音	53	投影	50	動脈硬化〔症〕	62
手首	136	盗汗	49	動脈瘤	62
手先具	28	動眼神経	117	透明性	42
手順書	42	動悸	50	投薬〔法〕	20
〔歩行保持用〕手すり	33	橈屈	3, 4	トウループ	33
手装具	29	橈屈外転	3	トーマススプリント(副子)	31
手継手	28	陶芸	23	トーマス免荷装具	30
鉄欠乏症	95	糖原病	102	兎眼	71
テニス肘	57	瞳孔〔の〕	122	トキソプラズマ	111
デニス-ブラウン装具	29	頭後屈反射	151	トキソプラズマ症	110
手背屈装具	29	統合失調型障害	107	〔中〕毒性ショック症候群	110
デュシェーヌ型筋ジス		統合失調感情障害	108	特定機能病院	38
トロフィー	58	統合失調症	108	禿頭〔症〕	74
手指義手	27	統合失調症様障害	108	禿頭の	123
てんかん	105	瞳孔反射	151	特発性の	48
転換性障害	105	橈骨〔の〕	137	特別養護老人ホーム	40
点眼薬	20	橈骨骨折	54	時計描画テスト	11
転帰	18	橈骨手根関節	137	吐血	48
電気刺激〔法〕	21	橈骨静脈	140	床ずれ	75
電気診断〔法〕	7	橈骨神経	139	徒手胸郭伸張法	25
デング熱	109	橈骨動脈	140	徒手筋力検査法	8
デング熱ウイルス	112	動作	25	突背	54
点字ブロック	34	籐細工	23	独歩	6, 60
〔ブライユ式〕点字法	32	同時失認	65	どもり	52
点耳薬	20	糖質代謝異常	96	ドライアイ症候群	70
点字用具	32	同時ひきずり歩行	60	トラコーマ	110
伝染性の	47	等尺性収縮	59	トランキライザー	110
点滴〔静注〕	21	豆状骨	137	トリコモナス症	110
転倒	5	同性愛	105	努力呼気量	10
電動義手	27	橈側手根屈筋	138	トルコ鞍	115
電動車椅子	33	頭長筋	116	トレッドミル試験	9
電動点字タイプライター	32	頭頂骨	115	ドロップ〔リング〕ロック	32
伝導熱療法	22	等張性収縮	59	トロント装具	29
転倒発作	44	疼痛	50	貪食細胞	146
天然痘	110	疼痛性障害	106		
殿部	141	〔真性〕糖尿病	92	**な**	
天疱瘡	76	頭髪	124	ナイアシン	153

ナイアシン欠乏症	95	
内果	141	
内耳	121	
内耳炎	73	
内耳孔	115	
内耳神経	117	
内旋	4	
内臓運動(感覚)神経	133	
内臓逆位症	102	
内臓神経	133	
内側広筋	144	
内腹斜筋	133	
内側直筋	116	
内側翼突筋	116	
内転	3	
内転筋	143	
内転筋結節	143	
内反	4	
内反膝	56	
内反尖足歩行	59	
内反〔尖〕足	56, 57	
内閉鎖筋	133	
内肋間筋	128	
ナックルベンダー	32	
ナルコレプシー	67	
軟骨形成不全症	54	
軟性コルセット	31	
軟性装具	29	
難聴	72	

に

にきび	74
肉腫	146
二次性の	51
二次的救命処置	17
二段呼吸	24
日常生活動作	4
日常生活動作テスト	9
日常生活動作評価尺度	15
日常生活満足度	15
日常生活用具	33
日光恐怖症	75

二点一点歩行	60
二点識別覚	13
二頭筋反射	150
二の腕	136
二分脊椎〔症〕	103
乳がん	87
乳児〔性〕〔の〕	49, 89
乳腺	135
乳腺炎	87
乳糖	153
乳頭筋	130
乳糖不耐症	95
乳〔様〕突〔起〕炎	72
乳房	128
乳房炎	87
乳房痛	87
乳様突起	115
入浴	25
入浴動作	4
ニューラプラキシア	67
乳〔汁〕漏〔出〕症	92
ニューロパチー	67
尿〔の〕	149
尿管〔の〕	135
尿管異所開口	84
尿管結石	86
尿細管	135
尿細管壊死	86
尿酸	153
尿酸代謝異常	96
尿失禁	86
尿〔結〕石	86
尿道	135
尿道炎	86
尿道括約筋	133
尿道狭窄	86
尿道症候群	86
尿道腟括約筋	133
尿毒症	86
尿崩症	84
尿路カンジダ症	86
尿路感染症	86

尿路結石症	86
人間ドック	7
妊娠	89
認知行動療法	22
認知症	105
認知障害	104
認知症評価尺度	12
認知不能〔症〕	64
認知リハビリテーション	35

ね

寝汗	49
猫背	54
寝たきり度	14
熱気浴	25
熱傷	74
ネフローゼ	85
ネフローゼ症候群	85
眠気	51
粘液〔性〕〔の〕	49
捻挫	57
捻転性(ねじれ)失調〔症〕	58
捻髪音	45
粘膜〔の〕	49

の

脳炎	65
脳外傷	66
脳幹	119
脳灌流圧	147
脳血管障害	65
脳血栓〔症〕	65
脳梗塞〔症〕	65
脳挫傷	65
脳腫瘍	65
脳循環	147
脳症	65
脳神経	117
膿腎症	85
脳震盪	65
脳性麻痺簡易運動検査	8
脳脊髄炎	66

脳塞栓〔症〕	65	背側の	125	発汗	50
脳卒中	66	肺動脈	129	薄筋	144
能動義手	27	肺動脈弁	129	白血球	146
脳内出血	65	肺動脈幹	129	白血球減少(増多)症	98
膿尿	85	梅毒	110	白血病	97
脳波検査〔法〕	7	排尿〔する〕	52, 149	発声障害	73
囊胞性腎疾患	84	排尿筋	132	発達指数	14
囊胞性線維症	102	排尿訓練	24	発達障害	105
脳梁	120	排尿困難	84	発熱	47
のど	131	排尿障害	86	発話障害	66
喉仏	131	排尿痛	84	鼻〔の〕	122
伸び上がり歩行	60	排尿反射	151	鼻茸	73
ノルアドレナリン	153	肺粘性抵抗	10	鼻血	73
ノルエピネフリン	153	背部痛	54	鼻ポリープ	73
ノロウイルス	112	ハイブリッドタイプ義手	27	鼻水	51
		ハイブリッドタイプ膝	28	パニック障害	106
は		排便	149	ハノイの塔	13
歯〔の〕	123	肺胞〔の〕	131	ハムストリング	144
パーキンソン病	65	肺胞換気	148	ハムストリング損傷	58
バーグ・バランス尺度	7	背面の	125	バラ疹	76
パーセント(%)肺活量	10	肺理学療法	21	パラチフス	110
ハーネス	27	ハイリスクパーソン	41	パラフィン浴	25
バーンアウト〔シンドローム〕	104	パイロン義足	28	腫れ	47
肺〔の〕	131	吐き気	49	破裂	59
肺〔臓〕炎	78	歯茎	123	ハロー装具	29
肺炎連鎖球菌	111	白質	121	斑	50
背臥位	2	剥奪	46	半陰陽	102
徘徊する	53	白内障	70	半球	120
肺活量	10	白斑	76	半月板	142
肺活量計	10	白皮症	101	反抗挑戦性障害	106
肺がん	78	麦粒腫	71	瘢痕	51
肺気腫	78	はげ	74	半昏睡	51
肺機能	149	跛行	5	半座位	2
肺気量	10	箱作り法	23	反射	150
背屈	4	箱庭療法	22	ハンセン病	109
敗血症	110	はさみ歩行	60	半側臥位	2
肺血栓塞栓症	79	はしか	110	反跳現象	51
肺コンプライアンス	10	梯子	33	反応	150, 152
肺水腫	79	把持装具	30	晩発性小脳皮質萎縮症	65
排泄動作	5	破傷風	110	晩発性の	52
背側骨間筋	138, 143	破水	89	反復唾液嚥下テスト	8
肺塞栓〔症〕	79	バチェラー〔型〕装具	30		

ひ

項目	ページ
BCGワクチン	22
PTES式下腿義足	30
PTB免荷装具	30
鼻咽頭炎	73
鼻炎	74
ビオプテリン代謝異常症	101
日帰り介護	37
皮下出血	48
光恐怖〔症〕	71
引き下げ	3
鼻筋	116
鼻腔	122
非経口〔的〕栄養〔補給〕	20
非結核性抗酸菌症	110
鼻孔	122
腓骨〔の〕	142
尾骨〔の〕	132
尾骨角	132
尾骨神経	133
鼻根筋	116
膝	141
膝折れ	5
膝がしら〔の〕	142
膝関節	142
膝義足	28
膝屈曲義足	28
膝屈筋〔群〕	144
膝クローヌス	56
膝装具	30
膝立位	2
〔安全〕膝継手	32
肘	136
肘関節	136
肘義手	27
肘装具	29
肘台付杖	32
皮質	119
肘継手	27
肘這い	5
肘反射	152
鼻出血	73
脾静脈	133
皮疹	75
非ステロイド抗炎症薬	19
鼻性反射神経症	73
鼻癤	73
鼻前庭	122
脾臓〔の〕	146
額	114
肥大	61
肥大型心筋症	61
非対称性緊張性頸反射	150
ビタミン	153
ビタミン過剰症	94
ビタミンA欠乏症	96
ビタミンC欠乏症	96
ビタミンD欠乏症	94
左手利きの	149
鼻中隔	122
鼻中隔弯曲症	74
必須脂肪酸欠乏症	94
必須の	47
ヒップサポーター	31
ビデオ造影検査〔法〕	9
ビデオ内視鏡検査〔法〕	9
脾動脈	133
ヒト免疫不全ウイルス	112
――感染症	90
ひとり歩き	6
微熱	47
皮膚〔の〕	123, 146
皮膚萎縮	74
皮膚壊死	75
皮膚炎	75
腓腹	141
腓腹筋	144
腓腹筋群	143
腓腹神経	145
皮膚硬化	76
皮膚紅痛症	75
皮膚症	75
飛蚊症	71
肥満〔症〕	95
びまん性軸索損傷	66
びまん(瀰漫)性の	46
紐づくり	23
冷や汗	45
百日咳	110
日焼け	52
ヒヤリハット報告	41
病院	38
評価	13, 14
描画テスト	12
病気	46, 48
表在性温熱療法	22
標準失語症検査	9
病訴	45
病態失認〔症〕	64
病的賭博	106
評点	16
病棟	38
表皮〔の〕	123
病歴	17
ヒラメ筋	144
びらん	51
鼻稜	115
ビリルビン尿	44
鼻漏	51
疲労感	47
疲労骨折	54
ピロゴフ切断	18
貧血	97
頻呼吸	79
頻尿〔症〕	85
頻発月経	87
頻脈	62

ふ

項目	ページ
ファウラー位	2
不安	44
不安障害	104
フィードバック	41

不育症	89	副鼻腔	123	分類不能型免疫不全症	91
部位誤認手術	42	副鼻腔炎	74		
風疹	110	腹壁反射	150	**へ**	
プール熱	110	腹膜炎	82	平均前腕装具	29
フェイルセーフの	41	服薬指導	20	平均棒訓練	24
フェニルケトン尿症	95	ふくらはぎ	141	閉経	87
フォークオーター切断	18	不随運動	60	閉鎖〔症〕	44
フォールトトレランス	41	不正咬合	82	閉鎖骨折	54
フォンローゼン装具	31	不正〔子宮〕出血	88	閉鎖神経	145
不快感	46	不整脈	61	閉塞性換気障害	78
ぷかぷか装具	30	不全	47	ペグボード	23
腹〔部〕〔の〕	132	不全対麻痺	68	臍〔の〕	132
腹圧	149	不全麻痺	68	ヘモグロビン血症	97
腹横筋	133	不全リンパ球症候群	91	ヘモクロマトーシス	63
腹臥位	2	腹筋	132	ペラグラ	95
複合運動活動電位	7	物〔理〕療〔法〕医学	35	弁	130
副睾丸炎	87	不動化	59	偏位	3
複合筋活動電位	7	ブドウ球菌〔の〕	111	〔大脳〕辺縁系	120
副甲状腺	114	不同視	70	変形	46
副甲状腺機能亢進症	93	ブドウ糖	152	変形性関節症	56
副甲状腺機能低下症	93	舞踏病	66	変形性骨炎	55
副甲状腺ホルモン	153	ブドウ膜炎	71	変形性脊椎炎	55
伏在静脈	145	不妊〔症〕	89	偏見	41
伏在神経	145	部分浴	25	片(偏)頭痛	65
複雑骨折	54	踏みきり	5	変性〔症〕	46
複視	70	不眠〔症〕	108	片側顔面れん(攣)縮	67
腹式呼吸	24, 149	ブライユ式点字法	32	片側骨盤用義足	28
福祉事務所	40	フラジャイルエックス症候群	102	片側性透過性亢進肺	79
福祉保健事務所	40	プラスチック装具	29	ベンダーゲシュタルト検査	12
輻射熱療法	22	ブルンストロームステージ	16	便通薬	20
副神経	117	フレンケル体操	24	〔口蓋〕扁桃炎	74
副腎酵素欠損症	101	ブローカ中枢(野)	119	扁桃肥大	52
副腎腫瘍	92	フロマン徴候	67	便秘	80
副腎性器症候群	92	プロラクチン産生腺腫	94	扁平足	56
副腎皮質過形成	92	分泌物	46	片麻痺	67
副腎皮質刺激ホルモン	153	分娩〔期〕	88, 89	**ほ**	
副腎皮質ステロイド薬	19	分回し	3	保育施設	39
副腎皮質不全(機能低下症)	92	分回し歩行	59	保育所	39
腹水	44	噴門〔の〕	134	ボイド切断	18
腹直筋	133	分類	13	包括的リハビリテーション	35
腹痛	80				

棒クレンザック	29	勃起障害	87	慢性閉塞性肺疾患	78
棒訓練	24	発作	44	**み**	
方形回内筋	139	発疹	75	ミエログラフィー	8
膀胱	134	発疹チフス	111	ミオクローヌス	67
膀胱炎	84	発赤	75	味覚	148
膀胱がん	84	ホットパック	25	右手利きの	149
膀胱乳頭がん	84	ボツリヌス菌	111	眉間	115
放散痛	50	ボツリヌス症	109	未熟児	88
放射線療法	21	歩幅	5	水治療法	21
胞状奇体	87	母斑〔症〕	76, 103	水飲みテスト	7
傍脊柱筋	126	頬	114	水ぼうそう	111
疱瘡	110	頬髭	124	水虫	76
蜂巣炎	74	ホモシスチン尿症	102	みぞおち	128
包帯	34	ポリープ	50	三日はしか	110
乏尿〔症〕	85	ポリオ	68	ミネソタ多面人格目録	12
包皮	124	ホルモン	153	耳詰まり	73
方法	15	本義肢	26	耳鳴り	72
膨満感	44	本態性の	47	脈絡膜炎	70
訪問看護	37	ポンポン	132	**む**	
訪問リハビリテーション	37	**ま**		無関心	64
ホームヘルパー	35	マイクロ波療法	21	無ガンマグロブリン血症	97
保健所	40	マクラメ	23	無嗅覚	73
歩行	5, 6, 59	マクログロブリン血症	99	むくみ	47
歩行器	33	マクロファージ	146	無月経	87
歩行障害	59	麻疹	110	無虹彩	101
歩行速度	5	麻酔薬	19, 20	無呼吸	78
歩行動作	4	まつげ	122	ムコ多糖〔体蓄積〕症	95
歩行補助杖	32	マッサージ	25	無言症	106
歩行率	5	末梢神経障害	67	無酸素性運動	24
母指(趾)	136, 141	末端肥大症	74	無酸素性作業閾値	16
母趾外転筋	143	松葉杖	32	霧視	71
母指球筋	139	松葉杖歩行	59	虫歯	82
母指探しテスト	9	麻痺	67	胸やけ	48
母子生活支援施設	40	麻薬	20	無毛〔性〕の	124
母指対立筋	139	眉〔毛〕	122	**め**	
母指(趾)内転筋	138, 143	マラスムス	95	目；眼〔の〕	122
ホスピス	38	満月状(様)顔〔貌〕	95	迷走神経	117
母性	89	慢性腎臓病	84	メープルシロップ尿症	103
保存療法	22	慢性肉芽腫症	91	メタボリックシンドローム	95
歩調	5	慢性の	45		
歩長	5	慢性疲労症候群	66		
補聴器	33				

メッツ；メット	15	薬剤事故	41	腰痛体操	24
メニエール病	67	薬疹	75	陽電子放出断層撮影〔法〕	8
メニスクス	142	薬物	20	腰部	125
めまい〔眩暈〕	52	薬物依存	105	腰方形筋	133
目脂	71	薬物有害事象	41	抑うつ〔症〕	105
メラノーマ	76	薬物乱用	44	抑うつ状態	105
免疫グロブリン	153	やけど	74	予後	18
免疫不全症	91	やすり磨き	23	予診	17
免疫療法	21	やせ病	96	〔出産〕予定日	89

も

		夜尿〔症〕	44	予備吸気量	10
		盲〔症〕	70	予備呼気量	10
盲	70			予防接種	22
毛根	124			よろめき歩き	6
毛細〔血〕管	129	## ゆ		四点(四脚)杖	32
盲児施設	39			四点歩行	59
妄想	105	有鈎骨	137		
〔持続性〕妄想性障害	105	疣贅	77	## ら	
盲腸	134	優先順位	41		
盲点	122	有毛〔性〕の	124	ライ症候群	65
毛髪	124	幽門〔の〕	134	ライソゾーム病	93
網膜〔の〕	122	有料老人ホーム	40	ラ音	51
網膜症	71	指〔の〕	136	ラセーグ徴候	16
網膜静脈；網膜動脈	118	指装具	29	卵円孔	115
盲・ろう児施設	39	指叩き試験	8	卵管	135
燃え尽き症候群	104	指の深静脈	140	卵管炎	88
モジュラー義肢	26	指鼻指テスト	8	乱視	70
モジュラー義足	28			卵子〔の〕	135
木工	23	## よ		卵巣〔の〕	135
物語に基づいた医療	17			卵巣炎	88
ものもらい	71	癰	74	卵巣がん	88
股義足	28	葉	120	卵巣機能障害	88
もやもや病	67	要介護認定	37	乱用	44
問診	17	胸棘筋	126		
門脈圧亢進症	82	葉酸	152	## り	
		腰三角	128		
## や		葉酸欠乏症	94	リーチャー	33
		腰神経；腰神経叢	127	リーメンビューゲル	32
野	119	羊水	134	リウマチ	57
夜間頻尿〔症〕	85	腰髄	127	リウマチ性多〔発性〕筋痛〔症〕	58
夜間用副子	31	妖精様顔〔貌〕症候群	103		
野球肘	56	腰仙椎装具	31	リウマチ熱	110
夜驚症	106	腰仙部挫傷	55	理学療法	21
薬剤	20	腰腸肋筋	126	理学療法士	35
		腰椎装具	31	リクライニング型車椅子	33
		腰痛	54		

リケッチア	111	リンパ管拡張症	98	裂孔ヘルニア	81
梨状筋	133	リンパ球	146	レット症候群	107
離人症障害	105	リンパ球減少	49	レム睡眠	148
リソソーム病	93	リンパ腫	99, 146	レム睡眠行動障害	107
立位	2	リンパ節	129	連合運動	60
立位保持装具	29	リンパ節炎	98	連合線維	119
立体認知	52	リンパ節結核	98	連鎖球菌〔の〕	111
立方骨	142	リンパ節症	98	攣縮	51
利尿薬	20	リンパ増殖症候群	99	連珠毛	103

リハビリテーション 35
── カウンセリング 37
リハビリテーション医 36
リハビリテーション工学 35
流行性耳下腺炎 109
流行性の 47
流産 88
隆椎 115
療育 21
良肢位 2
良性の 44
両手利き 149
療法 22
両麻痺 66
療養型病床群 38
療養型病棟 38
緑内障 71
淋疾 87
輪状甲状筋 115
臨床心理士 35
輪状軟骨 131
リンパ管 129
リンパ管異常 98
リンパ管炎 98

リンパ組織球増多症 99
リンパ肉腫 99
リンパ嚢腫 99
リンパ浮腫 99
リンパ脈管筋腫症 78
淋病 87

る

類鼾音 51
類癌腫 146
涙骨 115
涙腺 122
るいそう 94
涙道閉塞症(狭窄) 71
涙嚢 122
涙嚢炎 70
類白血病反応 98

れ

ルーケンベルグ切断 18
レクリエーション療法 22
レジスタンス運動 25
裂〔溝〕 47
裂肛 80

ろ

ろう(聾) 72
ろう学校 40
老眼 71
老視 71
ろう児施設 39
老人福祉センター 40
老年〔性〕の 51
ローテーターカフ 137
ロールシャッハテスト 12
ローレンツ固定装具 29
肋間隙 128
肋骨〔の〕 128

わ

歪曲視 71
若木骨折 54
腋 128
ワクチン 22
鷲手 45
腕神経叢 139
腕神経叢障害 66
腕橈骨筋 138

INDEX (英語索引)

A

abdomen; abdominal 132
abdominal breathing
　(respiration) 24, 149
abdominal muscle 132
abdominal pain 80
abdominal pressure 149
abdominal reflex 150
abducent nerve 117
abduction 3
abductor [muscle] 138
abductor digiti minimi
　[muscle] 138, 143
abductor hallucis [muscle]
　143
abductor pollicis brevis
　[muscle] 138
abductor pollicis longus
　[muscle] 138
abnormal heart rhythm 61
abnormal posture 2
abortion 88
above elbow (AE) amputation 18
above elbow prosthesis 27
above knee (AK) amputation 18
above knee prosthesis 28
abuse 44
acalasia 80
acalculia 64
acariasis 109
acarinosis 109
accessory nerve 117
accountability 41
acetabulum 132
ache 50
Achilles tendon 141
　—— reflex (ATR) 150
　—— rupture 59
achillobursitis 55

achondroplasia 54
acidosis 44
acne 74
acoustic reaction 11
acoustic trauma 72
acoustic tumor 72
acquired 44
acquired immunodeficiency
　syndrome (AIDS) 90
acrocephalopolysyndactyly 101
acromegalic gigantism 92
acromegaly 92
acromion 136
action potential 7
active assistive exercise
　(movement) 24
active movement 25
activities of daily living (ADL) 4
　—— Scale 15
activities parallel to daily
　living (APDL) 4
acute 44
acute hospital 38
acute phase rehabilitation 35
acute stress disorder
　(ASD) 104
Adam's apple 120
addiction 44
adduction 3
adductor [muscle] 143
adductor brevis [muscle] 132
adductor hallucis [muscle]
　143
adductor longus [mus-cle]
　132
adductor magnus [muscle]
　132
adductor pollicis [muscle] 138
adductor tubercle 143
adenoid[al] hypertrophy 48

adenosine deaminase
　(ADA) deficiency 101
adiposity 94
adjunctive [walking] stick 32
adjustment disorder 104
adrenal enzyme deficiency 101
adrenal tumor 92
adrenaline 152
adrenocortical hyperplasia 92
adrenocortical insufficiency 92
adrenocorticosteroid 19
adrenocorticotropic
　hormone (ACTH) 153
adrenogenital syndrome
　(AGS) 92
adult respiratory distress
　syndrome (ARDS) 78
advanced life support
　(ALS) 17
adverse drug events 41
affective disorder 104
agammaglobulinemia 97
age-related macular
　degeneration (AMD) 71
agnosia 64
agoraphobia 104
agrammatism 64
agraphia 64
ailment 48
airway 131
albinism 101
alcohol rehabilitation
　program (ARP) 20
alcoholism 44, 104
aldosteronism 92
alexia 64
alkalosis 44
allergy; allergic 44
alopecia 74
alopecia areate 74

Term	Page
alternating three-point gait	59
alveolar arch	114
alveolar process	114
alveolar ventilation	148
alveolitis	82
alveolus; alveolar	131
Alzheimer dementia	105
Alzheimer disease	64
ambidexterity	149
amblyopia	70
ambulation activity	4
ambulatory rehabilitation (day care)	37
ameba; amebic	111
amenorrhea	87
amino acid	152
amnesia	104
amniorrhexis	89
amniotic fluid	134
amputation	18
amyloidosis	92
amyotrophic lateral sclerosis (ALS)	68
anacusis	72
anaerobics	24
anaerobics threshold (AT)	16
anal atresia	101
anal fissure	80
anal fistula	80
anal prolapse	80
anal sphincter	132
analgesic	19
anarthria	64
anatomical position	2
anconeus [muscle]	138
anemia	97
anesthetic	19
aneurysm	62
angi[i]tis	62
angina pectoris	61
aniridia	101
anisometropia	70
ankle	141
ankle bone	143
ankle foot orthosis (AFO)	30
ankylosing spondylitis	55
ankylosis	55
anorectic	19
anorexia	44, 104
anorexia nervosa	104
anosmia	73
anosognosia	64
anteflexion	4
anterior clinoid process	114
anterior cruciate ligament	142
anterior interosseous nerve	126
anterior longitudinal ligament	142
anterior standing position	2
anthrax	109
anti-inflammatory drug	19
antiallergic	19
antianxiety drug	19
antibiotic	19
antibody	153
anticoagulant	19
antidepressant	19
antidepressive agent	19
antidiarrheal	19
antidiuretic hormone (ADH)	153
antidote	19
antifebrile	20
antigen	152
antihistamine	19
antihyperlipidemic	19
antihypertensive	19
antiphospholipid antibody syndrome (APS)	90
antipyretic	20
antirheumatic drug	20
antithrombotic	19
antitussive	20
anus; anal	134
anxiety	44
anxiety disorder	104
anxiolytic	19
aorta; aortic	129
aortic aneurysm	62
aortic arch	129
aortic atresia	61
aortic insufficiency	61
aortic regurgitation	61
aortic valve	129
apathy	64
ape hand	69
apex cordis; apex of heart	130
aphasia	64
aphonia	64
apnea	78
aponeurotic reflex	150
appendicitis	80
appendix	134
appetite depressant	19
appetite suppressant	19
apraxia	64
aproctia	101
arachnoid [mater]	119
Arbeitsarm	27
arch of foot	141
area	119
arm	136
arm sling	32
armpit	128
arrhythmia	61
arse	141
art therapy	21
arteriosclerosis	62
arteritis	62
artery; arterial	129
arthralgia	55
arthritis	55
arthrodesis	18
arthrokinematic approach (AKA)	17
arthroplasty	18
arthrosis	56
articular contracture	56

articular deformity	56	
articulation disorder	65	
artificial insemination	89	
artificial joint replacement	18	
ascites	44	
aspirin	20	
ass	141	
assessment	13	
assistant dog	33	
associated movement	60	
association fiber	119	
astatic seizure	44	
asthenopia	70	
asthma	78	
astigmatism	70	
asymmetric tonic neck reflex (ATNR)	150	
ataxia	65	
atherosclerosis	62	
athetoid movement	60	
athetosis	66	
athlete's foot	76	
atlas	114	
atopic dermatitis	75	
atopic eczema	75	
atrial septal defect (ASD)	62	
atrium; atrial	130	
atrophia cutis	74	
atrophoderma	74	
atrophy	44	
attack	44	
attention-deficit / hyperactivity disorder (ADHD)	104	
audiometry	11	
audition	147	
auditory (hearing) acuity	147	
auditory agnosia	72	
auditory canal	121	
auditory fatigue	72	
auditory hallucination	72, 105	
auditory nerve	117	
auditory sensation area	147	
auditory threshold	147	

auricle	121, 130	
auscultation	17	
autism	104	
autogenic training	24	
autoimmune	44	
automated external defibrillator (AED)	20	
automatic walking	6	
axilla	128	
axillary cavity	128	
axillary nerve	129, 139	
axis	114	

B

Bacillus anthracis	111	
bacillus Calmette-Guérin (BCG) vaccine	22	
back	125	
back pain	54	
backbone	125	
backward elevation	3	
backward flexion	4	
bacterial food poisoning	109	
bacterium; bactrial	111	
balanced forearm orthosis (BFO)	29	
balanoposthitis	87	
bald	123	
baldness	74	
ball and socket ankle joint	141	
bandage	34	
bare lymphocyte syndrome	91	
basal blood pressure	7	
basal ganglia	119	
basal metabolic rate (BMR)	8	
baseball elbow	56	
basic activities of daily living (BADL)	4	
basic life support (BLS)	17	
Batchelor orthosis	30	
bath	25	

bathing activity	4	
bathroom	33	
beaded hair	103	
beard	123	
beating	25	
bed bath	25	
bed-wetting	44	
bedpan	34	
bedsore	75	
behavioral assessment	13	
belch	44	
belly	132	
belly button	132	
below elbow (BE) amputation	18	
below elbow prosthesis	27	
below knee (BK) amputation	18	
below-knee prosthesis	28	
Bender Gestalt Test	12	
bending	3	
benign	44	
bent knee prosthesis	28	
Berg Balance Scale	7	
beriberi	94	
bias	41	
biceps brachii [muscle]	138	
biceps femoris [muscle]	143	
biceps femoris reflex	150	
biceps muscle of thigh	143	
biceps reflex	150	
bicuspid [tooth]	123	
bicycle ergometer	32	
bilirubinuria	44	
biopterin metabolic disorder	101	
bipolar disorder	106	
bipolar hip arthroplasty	18	
birth weight	88	
birthmark	76	
bladder	134	
bladder cancer	84	
bladder papilloma	84	
bladder training	24	

bleeding	48	brain tumor	65	calvities	74
blepharoptosis	70	brain wave	7	calx	141
blind spot	122	brainstem	119	campimetry	11
blindness	70	breast	128	cancer	146
blink reflex	150	breast cancer	87	candida	111
blister	74	breathing	24	candidiasis	109
bloat[ing]	44	breathing exercise	23	cane	32
blood brain barrier	119	Broca center (area)	119	cane work	23
blood loss	45	bronchial ectasia	78	canine [tooth]	123
blood pressure	7	bronchiectasis	78	canker sore	82
blood pressure measurement	9	bronchiole; bronchiolar	131	canvas corset	31
bloody sputum	51	bronchitis	78	capillary	129
body (internal) powered prosthesis	26	bronchodilator	20	carbuncle	74
body dysmorphic disorder	104	bronchogenic carcinoma	78	carcinoid	146
body mass index (BMI)	13	bronchus; bronchial	131	carcinoid syndrome	92
body-powered upper limb prosthesis	27	bruise	45	carcinoma	146
boil	75	bruit	63	cardia; cardiac	134
bone conduction	11	Brunnstrom stage	16	cardiac	130
bottom	141	buccinator [muscle]	115	cardiac amyloidosis	61
bottom hitching	5	bucking	5	cardiac arrest	61
botulinum	111	bulimia nervosa	104	cardiac insufficiency	61
botulism	109	bulla	74	cardiac rehabilitation	35
bovine spongiform encephalopathy (BSE)	109	bullous keratopathy	71	cardiac tumor	61
bowel	134	burn [injury]	74	cardiomyopathy	61
bowel medicine	20	burning pain	50	cardiopulmonary resuscitation (CPR)	21
bowleg	56	burning sensation	45	care house	39
Boyd amputation	18	burnout syndrome	104	care management	37
brachial artery	140	burp	44	care manager	35
brachial plexopathy	66	bursitis	56	care worker	35
brachial plexus	139	buttocks	141	carious tooth	82
brachial vein	140	buttress	26	carotid arteries	118
brachial; brachial	136	**C**		carotid tubercle	114
brachialis [muscle]	138	C-bar	33	carpal tunnel	139
brachioradialis [muscle]	138	cadence	5	——— syndrome	66
bradycardia	61	cadence rate	5	carpometacarpal (CM) joint	136
braille	32	calcaneal gait	59	carpus; carpal	136
braille writing equipment	32	calcaneal reflex	150	case management	37
brain concussion	65	calcaneal tendon	141	case work	37
brain contusion	65	calcaneus; calcaneal	141	case worker	35
		calcification	45	cataplexy	66
		calf	141	cataract	70
		calf muscles	143		

catatonia	104	cervix [of uterus]	135	circumduction gait	59
CATCH22 syndrome	101	chair sitting position	2	cirrhosis	80
cathartic	20	CHARGE association		classification	13
causalgia	66	[syndrome]	101	claudication	5
cecum	134	checkup	7	clavicle; clavicular	136
celiac disease	80	cheek	114	claw foot	57
cellulitis	74	chemotherapy	21	clawhand	45
center	119	chest	128	cleft lip and palate	102
center of gravity	5	chest physical therapy	21	climacteric disturbance	87
central nerve	117	chickenpox	111	clinical assessment	13
central nervous system		chief complaint	45	clinical path	41
(CNS)	117	child guidance center	39	clinical psychologist	35
cephalalgia	48	child rearing facility	39	clitoris	135
ceramics	23	child welfare institution	39	Clock Drawing Test (CDT)	11
cerebellar arteries	118	childbirth	88	cloisonné	23
cerebellum; cerebellar	120	chills	45	closed fracture	54
cerebral infarction	65	chin	114	clubfoot	57
cerebral arteries	118	chin reflex	150	coordinate exercise	23
cerebral circulation	147	chlamydia; chlamydial	111	coordination test (Cord-T)	7
cerebral concussion	65	chloasma	74	coccus; coccal	111
cerebral contusion	65	choana	122	coccygeal cornu (horn)	132
cerebral embolism	65	cholangitis	80	coccygeal nerve	133
cerebral hemorrhage	65	cholecyst	134	coccyx; coccygeal	132
cerebral perfusion		cholecystitis	80	cochlea	121
pressure	147	choledocholithiasis	80	cochlear nerve	117
cerebral plasticity	147	cholelith[iasis]	80	cock-up splint	31
cerebral thrombosis	65	cholera	109	cognitive behavior therapy	22
cerebral tumor	65	cholesterol	152	cognitive disorder	104
cerebral veins	118	chorea	66	cognitive rehabilitation	35
cerebrospinal fluid (CSF)	147	choroiditis	70	[common] cold	45
cerebrovascular disorder		chromaffin cell tumor	93	cold medicine	20
(CVD)	65	chromatosis	76	cold remedy	20
cerebrum; cerebral	120	chromosomal syndrome	102	cold sore	109
certified social worker	36	chronic	45	cold sweat	45
cerumen	72	chronic fatigue syndrome		colic	45
cervical [spinal] cord	120	(CFS)	66	colitis	80
cervical canal stenosis	54	chronic glamnulomatous		collar bone	136
cervical cancer	87	disease (CGD)	91	collateral ligament	142
cervical cord injury	65	chronic kidney disease	84	colon	134
cervical nerve	117	chronic obstructive pulmonary		colon cancer	80
cervical orthosis	31	disease (COPD)	78	color blindness	70
cervical vertebrae	114	cilia	122	color sensation	147
cervix; cervical	114	circumduction	3	color vision defect	70

color vision deficiency	70	
coma	45	
commode chair	33	
common bile duct	134	
common iliac artery	133	
common iliac vein	133	
common peroneal (fibular) nerve	145	
common variable immunodeficiency	91	
communicating arteries	118	
communication	41	
community rehabilitation	37	
commuting care	37	
commuting rehabilitation service	37	
complaint	45	
complete checkup	7	
complex fracture	54	
complication	45	
compound fracture	54	
compound motor action potential	7	
compound muscle action potential	7	
compression bandage	34	
compression fracture	54	
computed tomography (CT)	7	
conduct disorder	104	
conductive heat therapy	22	
condyloma acuminatum	87	
confusion	45	
congenital	45	
congenital adrenal hyperplasia	102	
congenital defects	102	
congenital dislocation of hip joint	56	
congenital heart disease	102	
congenital hydronephrosis	102	
congenital insensitivity to pain with anhidrosis (CIPA)	102
congenital photomyoclonus	102
congestive heart failure (CHF)	61
conjugate gaze	147
conjugate movement of eyes	147
conjunctival reflex	150
conjunctivitis	70
consciousness clouding	45
conservative treatment	22
constipation	80
consultation office for children	39
contact dermatitis	75
continuative passive motion (CPM) therapy	22
continuous quality improvement (CQI)	41
contraction	59
contracture	45, 58
contrast bath	25
conventional lower limb prosthesis	28
conversion disorder	105
convulsion	45
coracobrachialis [muscle]	138
corneal reflex	150
corneal xerosis	70
coronary artery	129
coronary artery disease (CAD)	61
coronary heart disease (CHD)	61
coronavirus disease 2019 (COVID-19)	109
corpus callosum	120
corrective brace	34
corrective shoes	30
cortex	119
cosmetic prosthesis	26
cosmetic upper limb prosthesis	27
costa; costal	128
cough	45
cough medicine	20
cough reflex	150
coxal bone	132
crackle	45
cranial nerves	117
creeping	5
cremasteric reflex	150
crepitation	45
crepitus	45
CREST syndrome	56
Creutzfeldt-Jakob disease (CJD)	66
cricoid cartilage	131
cricothyroid [muscle]	115
crisis management	41
criteria	14
critical path	41
cross-eyed	70
crossed leg sitting position	2
crouching position	2
croup	78
cruciate ligament	142
crust	74
crutch	32
crutch gait	59
cuboid	142
Cushing disease	92
cuspid [tooth]	123
cuticle	123
cutis; cutaneous	124
cutout cushion	33
cyanosis	45
cystic fibrosis	102
cystic kidney disease	84
cystitis	84
cytomegalovirus (CMV)	112

D

Term	Page
dacryocystitis	70
dacryostenosis	71
daily living utensil	33
Damen korsett	31
dark adaptation	147
day blindness	70
day-care center	38
dead space	148
deafness	72
decubital ulcer	75
deep digital veins	140
deep heating therapy	22
deep palmar arch	140
deep peroneal (fibular) nerve	145
defecation	149
deficiency	46
deformity	46
degeneration	46
deglutition	148
degree of the bedridden	14
dehydration	46
delirium	105
delivery	88
deltoid [muscle]	138
deltoid reflex	150
delusion	105
[persistent] delusional disorder	105
dementia	105
dementia rating scale	12
dengue fever	109
dengue virus	112
Denis Browne orthosis	29
dens; dental	123
dental alveolus	114
dental caries	82
dental decay	82
dependence	46
depersonalization disorder	105
depigmentation	75
depressed fracture	54
depression	3, 105
depressive state	105
depressor	19
depressor anguli oris [muscle]	115
deprivation	46
derangement	46
dermatitis	75
dermatonecrosis	75
dermatosis	75
dermatrophia	74
dermis; dermal	123
derotation brace	32
detrusor [muscle]	132
developmental disability/disorder	105
developmental quotient	14
deviation	3
dextromanual	149
diabetes insipidus	84
diabetes mellitus	92
diagnosis	17
diagonal socket	26
diaper	33
diaphragm; diaphragmatic	128
diarrhea	80
didy	33
dietary calcium deficiency	94
difficulty in hearing	72
diffuse	46
diffuse axonal injury (DAI)	66
diffusion of responsibility	41
digestant	20
digestive	20
digestive tract (tube)	134
digit; digital	136
dilatation	46
dilated cardiomyopathy (DCM)	61
diphtheria	109
diplegia	66
diplopia	70
disability	46
disabled	46
disabled people (children)	36
disarticulation	18, 56
discharge	46
disclosure	41
discography	19
discoid meniscus	56
discomfort	46
disease	46
disinhibition	46
[intervertebral] disc herniation	54
dislocation	56
disorder	46
disorientation	46, 65
dissociative disorder	105
distal interphalangeal (DIP) joints	136
disturbance	46
disturbance in visual field	46
disturbance of consciousness	47
disturbance of memory	47
diuretic	20
dizziness	52
dorsal	125
dorsal interossei [muscle of foot]	143
dorsal interossei [muscle of hand]	138
dorsal position	2
dorsal root ganglion	127
dorsalis pedis artery	145
dorsiflexion	4
double vision	70
drawing test	12
dressing	25
dressing activity	4
drink test	7
drip	21

Term	Page
drop attack	44
drop foot	56
drop ring lock	32
dropsy	47
drowsiness	51
drug	20
drug abuse	44
drug administration guidance	20
drug dependence	105
drug eruption	75
dry eye syndrome	70
Duchenne muscular dystrophy (DMD)	58
due date	89
duodenal cancer	80
duodenal ulcer	80
duodenitis	80
duodenum; duodenal	134
dura [mater]	120
dwarfism	92
dysarthria	65
dyschromatopsia	70
dysentery	109
dysfunction	47
dyskinesia	59
dyslipidemia	94
dysmenorrhea	87
dysosmia	73
dyspepsia	82
dysphagia	80
dysphemia	52
dysphonia	73
dyspnea	78
dysthymic disorder	105
dystonia	58
dystonic movement	60
dystrophy	47
dysuria	84

E

Term	Page
ear discharge	72
ear drop	20
ear noise	72
ear pain	72
eardrum	121
earlobe	121
earwax	72
eating disorder	105
Ebola hemorrhagic fever	109
Ebola virus	112
echo; echography	9
ecstasy	47
ectopic ACTH syndrome	92
ectopic ossification	58
ectopic testis	102
ectopic ureter	84
eczema	75
edema	47
educational rehabilitation	35
effusion	47
elastosis	75
elbow	136
elbow disarticulation prosthesis	27
elbow joint	27, 136
elbow orthosis	29
elbow reflex	152
electric braille writer	32
electric upper limb prosthesis	27
electric wheelchair	33
electrical stimulation	21
electrocardiogram [-graphy] (ECG)	7
electrodiagnosis (EDX)	7
electroencephalogram [-graphy] (EEG)	7
electromyogram [-graphy] (EMG)	7
elephantiasis	97
elevation	3
elfin facies syndrome	103
emaciation	94
embolus	47
emergency room	38
emesis	52
emotional disorder	104
emotional lability	47
emphysema	78
Employees' Pension Fund (EPF)	37
encephalitis	65
encephalomyelitis	66
encephalopathy	65
endocarditis	61
endocardium	130
endometriosis	87
endoskeletal lower limb prosthesis	28
endoskeletal prosthesis	26
enteritis	80
enterobacterium	111
enterobiasis	109
enterocele	80
enzyme	152
epicranius [muscle]	115
epidemic	47
epidemic paroti[di]tis	109
epidemic typhus	111
epidermis; epidermal	123
epidermolysis bullosa hereditaria	102
epididymitis	87
epigastrium	128
epiglottic cartilage	131
epiglottis	131
epilepsy	105
epimenorrhea	87
epinephrine	152
epipharyngeal nerve	117
epipharyngitis	73
epistaxis	73
eponychium	136
equinovarus gait	59
equinus foot	57
erectile dysfunction	87
erector spinae [muscle]	126

ergometer	32	
eructation	44	
eruption	75	
erysipelas	109	
erythema	75	
erythralgia	75	
erythrocyte	146	
erythrocytosis	97	
erythrodema	76	
Escherichia coli	111	
esophageal carcinoma	80	
esophageal reflux	81	
esophageal varix	63	
esophagitis	81	
esophagus; esophageal	134	
essential	47	
essential fatty acid deficiency	94	
ethmoid [bone]	114	
ethmoidal labyrinth	114	
euphoria	105	
eustachian tube	121	
evaluation	14	
eversion	3	
everyday memory checklist	12	
evidence-based medicine (EBM)	17	
exarticulation	56	
exchange handedness	23	
exercise	24	
exercise electrocardiography	7	
exercise for low back pain	24	
exercise prescription	18	
exophthalmos	70	
exoskeletal prosthesis	26	
expiration	148	
expiratory muscle	128	
expiratory reserve volume (ERV)	10	
extension	3	
extensor carpi radialis brevis [muscle]	138	
extensor carpi radialis longus [muscle]	138	
extensor carpi ulnaris [muscle]	138	
extensor digiti minimi [muscle]	138	
extensor digitorum brevis [muscle]	143	
extensor digitorum longus [muscle]	143	
extensor digitorum muscle	138	
extensor hallucis brevis [muscle]	143	
extensor hallucis longus [muscle]	143	
extensor indicis [muscle]	138	
extensor pollicis brevis [muscle]	138	
extensor pollicis longus [muscle]	138	
external acoustic (auditory) meatus	121	
external acoustic (auditory) pore	114	
external ear	121	
external intercostal [muscle]	128	
external oblique [muscle]	132	
—— reflex	150	
external otitis	73	
external powered prosthesis	26	
external rotation	4	
extraocular muscles	116	
extrapyramidal [motor] system	120	
extremely immature infant	88	
eye	122	
eye chart	11	
eye drop	20	
eye examination	10	
eye mucus	71	
eyeball	122	
eyebrow	122	
eyelashes	122	
eyesight test	11	
—— chart	11	
eyestrain	70	

F

face flush	47
facial nerve	117
facial reflex	150
facility	38
fail-safe	41
failure	47
faint	47
faintness	47
fall	5
Fallopian tube	135
familial	47
familial polyposis coli (FPC)	102
family history	17
far-sightedness	71
fatigue	47
fatigue fracture	54
fatty acid	152
fatty liver	81
faucial reflex	150
fault-tolerance	41
feedback	41
feeding activity	4
femoral artery	145
femoral neck	142
—— fracture	54
femoral nerve	145
femoral vein	145
femur; femoral	141, 142
fertilization	89
fetus; fetal	89
fever	47
fever blister	109
fibrodysplasia ossificans progressiva	102

fibula; fibular	142	
fibularis brevis [muscle]	143	
fibularis longus [muscle]	143	
fibularis tertius [muscle]	143	
field of vision	147	
finding	47	
finger	136	
finger orthosis	29	
finger prosthesis	27	
finger tapping test	8	
finger to nose to finger test	8	
fingerprint	136	
first evaluation	14	
fissure	47	
fist	136	
fit	44, 45	
flank	132	
flank pain	81	
flatfoot	57	
flexion	3	
flexion reflex	150	
flexor carpi radialis [muscle]	138	
flexor carpi ulnaris [muscle]	138	
flexor digiti minimi brevis [muscle]	138, 144	
flexor digitorum brevis [muscle]	144	
flexor digitorum longus [muscle]	144	
flexor digitorum profundus [muscle]	138	
flexor digitorum superficialis [muscle]	138	
flexor hallucis brevis [muscle]	144	
flexor hallucis longus [muscle]	144	
flexor pollicis brevis [muscle]	138	
flexor pollicis longus [muscle]	139	
flexor reflex	151
flu	110
flying flies	71
focal motor seizure	66
folic acid	152
folic acid deficiency	94
folie à deux	108
foot	141
foot-and-mouth disease (FMD)	109
foot flat	5
footdrop	56
foramen magnum	114
foramen ovale	115
forced expiratory volume (FEV)	10
forced vital capacity (FVC)	10
forearm	136
forehead	114
foreign body	47
forequarter amputation	18
foreskin	124
forming with coils	23
forward elevation	3
forward flexion	4
four-legged cane	32
four-point gait	59
Fowler position	2
fracture (Frx)	54
fragile X syndrome	102
frame corset	31
Frenkel exercise	24
frequent urination	85
Froment sign	67
frontal bone	115
frontalis [muscle]	116
frozen shoulder	57
fulminant	47
fulminating	47
fumeral fracture	54
functional dead space	148
functional electrical stimulation (FES)	21

Functional Independence Measure (FIM)	8
functional occupational therapy	22
functional position	2
functional rehabilitation training	24
functional residual capacity (FRC)	10
functional training	24
functional upper limb prosthesis	27
fundamental position	2
fundus examination	10
funduscopy	10
fungus	111
furuncle	75
furunculosis	75

G

gag reflex	151
gait	5, 59
gait disturbance	59
gait on heels	59
gait velocity	5
galactorrhea	92
gallbladder	134
gallbladder cancer	81
gangliated cord	121
ganglion	58
gangrene	48
gape	53
gas exchange	148
gastric	134
gastric cancer	81
gastric diverticulum	81
gastric hyperacidity	81
gastric subacidity	81
gastric ulcer	81
gastritis	81
gastrocnemius [muscle]	144
gastroenteritis	81
gastroenteropathy	81

gastroesophageal reflux disease (GERD)	81	
gastroptosis	81	
Gatch bed	33	
gaze	147	
general malaise	48	
generic drug	20	
genioglossus [muscle]	116	
geniohyoid [muscle]	116	
genital herpes	87	
genu	141	
genu valgum	56	
genu varum	56	
germ	111	
gestation	89	
gibbus	54	
gigantism	93	
gingiva; gingival	123	
gingival bleeding	82	
gingivitis	82	
Gips	34	
Gipsschiene	34	
glabella	115	
Glasgow Coma Scale (GCI)	15	
glaucoma	71	
glenohumeral joint	136	
glioma	67	
glomerulonephritis	84	
glomerulus; glomerular	135	
glossitis	82	
glossopharyngeal nerve	117	
glottis	131	
glucose	152	
gluten enteropathy	80	
gluteus maximus [muscle]	144	
—— gait	59	
gluteus medius [muscle]	144	
—— gait	60	
gluteus minimus [muscle]	144	
glycogenosis	102	
gonadotropic hormone	153	
gonadotropin	153	

gonadotropin-releasing hormone (GRH, GnRH)	153	
gonorrhea	87	
gout	94	
gouty tophus	48	
gracilis [muscle]	144	
gray matter	120	
great toe	141	
greater trochanter	142	
greater tubercle (tuberosity)	142	
green stick fracture	54	
grip strength	8	
grippe	110	
groin	132	
grooming activity	4	
group home	39	
group training	24	
growth	48, 146	
growth hormone	153	
gum	123	
gut	134	

H

habilitation	21	
hair	124	
hair root	124	
hairless	124	
hairy	124	
half kneeling	5	
half side-lying position	2	
half-sitting position	2	
hallucination	105	
halo brace (orthosis)	29	
hamate	137	
hamstring [muscles]	144	
—— injury	58	
hand	136	
hand dorsal orthosis	29	
hand-foot-and-mouth disease (HFMD)	109	
hand joint	137	
hand orthosis	29	

hand-rail and support rail	33	
handicap	48	
Hansen disease	109	
harness	27	
head	114	
head retraction reflex	151	
headache	48	
hearing	147	
hearing impairment	72	
hearing loss	72	
hearing-aid	33	
heart	130	
heart attack	62	
heart failure	61	
heart rate	8	
heartburn	48	
heavy chain disease	97	
heel	141	
heel bumper	32	
height	8	
heliophobia	75	
hematemesis	48	
hematospermia	87	
hematuria	84	
hemeralopia	70	
hemifacial spasm	67	
hemipelvectomy prosthesis	28	
hemiplegia	67	
hemisphere	120	
hemochromatosis	63	
hemoglobinemia	97	
hemophilia	97	
hemorrhage	48	
hemorrhagic fever	109	
hemorrhoid	81	
hepatic	134	
hepatic blood flow	149	
hepatic failure	81	
hepatitis	81	
hepatocarcinoma	81	
hepatocellular carcinoma (HCC)	81	
hepatomegaly	81	

hepatopathy	81	
hereditary	48	
heredoataxia	102	
hermaphroditism	102	
herniated disc	54	
herpes genitals	87	
herpes labials	109	
herpes simplex	109	
── virus (HSV)	112	
herpes zoster	110	
heterosexuality	105	
heterotaxia	102	
heterotropia	71	
hiatal hernia	81	
hiccup	48	
high blood pressure	63	
high fever	47	
high risk person	41	
High-cost Medical Care Benefits	37	
higher brain dysfunction	65	
hindfoot	141	
hip	125	
hip bone	132	
hip joint	132	
hip orthosis	30	
hip prosthesis	28	
hip supporter	31	
hip-knee-ankle-foot orthosis (HKAFO)	30	
hippocampus; hippocampal		120
hirsuitism	75	
histiocytosis	97	
[medical] history	17	
hives	77	
hoarseness	48	
holistic rehabilitation	35	
home helper	35	
home making (house-work) activity	5	
home rehabilitation	37	
homocystinuria	102	
homosexuality	105	
hop on one leg	5	
hordeolum	71	
horizontal abduction	3	
horizontal adduction	3	
horizontal extension	3	
horizontal flexion	3, 4	
hormone	153	
hospice	38	
hospital	38	
hospital home for physically handicapped children	39	
hospital-acquired infection		110
hot air bath	25	
hot pack	25	
House-Tree-Person (HTP) Test	12	
Hubbard tank	32	
human error	41	
human immunodefi-ciency virus (HIV)	112	
── infection	90	
humerus; humeral	137	
humpback	54	
hunchback	54	
hyaloid body	122	
hybrid type knee	28	
hybrid type prosthesis	27	
hydatidiform mole	87	
hydrocephalus	102	
hydronephrosis	84	
hydrotherapy	21	
hyoid bone	115	
hyperalimentation	21	
hypercalcemia	94	
hypercholesterolemia	94	
hyperemia	48	
hyperimmunogloblin E syndrome	91	
hyperkalemia	94	
hyperkinetic disorder	105	
hyperlipidemia	94	
hypermetropia	71
hyperopia	71
hyperparathyroidism	93
hyperpathia	48
hyperphagia	107
hyperpituitarism	93
hyperplasia	146
hyperpotassemia	94
hypertension	63
hyperthermia	48
hyperthyroidism	93
hypertrichosis	75
hypertrophic cardiomyopathy (HCM)	61
hypertrophy	48
hyperuricemia	94
hyperventilation syndrome	78
hypervitaminosis	94
hypnotic	20
hypocalcemia	94
hypochondria	105
hypochondriasis	105
hypogastalgia	82
hypoglossal nerve	117
hypoglycemia	48
hypokalemia	95
hypoparathyroidism	93
hypophysis	120
hypopituitarism	93
hypopotassemia	95
hypoproteinemia	95
hyposmia	73
hypotension	63
hypothalamus; hypothalamic	120
hypothenar muscle	139
hypothermia	48
hypothyroidism	93

I

ice massage	25
Icelandic roll-on silicone socket (ICEROSS)	26

255

ichthyosis vulgaris	76	
identity disorder	105	
idiopathic	48	
ileum; ileal	134	
ileus	82	
iliacus [muscle]	132	
iliocostalis cervicis [muscle]	126	
iliocostalis lumborum [muscle]	126	
iliocostalis thoracis [muscle]	126	
iliopsoas [muscle]	133	
iliotibial tract	142	
ilium; iliac	132	
illness	48	
immature infant	88	
immobilization	59	
immunodeficiency	91	
immunoglobulin	153	
immunotherapy	21	
impairment	48	
implant; implantation	19	
impotence	87	
in vitro fertilization (IVF)	89	
in-home care	37	
in-home [welfare] services	37	
inappropriate ADH syndrome	93	
inappropriate prolactin syndrome	93	
incontinence	49	
incus	115	
independent gait	60	
index	15	
indigestion	82	
industrial disease	17	
infant; infantile	49, 89	
infantile	49	
infarct; infarction	49	
infection; infectious	49	
infective	49	

inferior constrictor [muscle] of pharynx	116	
inferior gemellus [muscle]	144	
infertility	89	
inflammation	49	
inflammatory	49	
inflammatory bowel disease (IBD)	82	
influenza	110	
informed consent	17	
infrared treatment	21	
infraspinatus [muscle]	126	
infusion	21	
inguinal hernia	82	
inguinal region	132	
injection	21	
injector	21	
inoculation	21	
insemination	89	
insomnia	108	
inspection	17	
inspiration	148	
inspiratory capacity	10	
inspiratory reserve volume (IRV)	10	
instep	141	
institution for severely retarded children	38	
insulin	153	
intellectual impairment	106	
intelligence quotient	15	
intelligibility of speech	11	
intercarpal joints	137	
intercostal space	128	
intermittent	49	
intermittent claudication	5, 60	
internal acoustic opening	115	
internal ear	121	
internal intercostal [muscle]	128	
internal oblique [muscle]	133	
internal otitis	73	

internal rotation	4	
intertarsal joint	142	
intervertebral disc	125	
—— herniation	54	
intervertebral foramen	125	
intervertebral joint	125	
intestinal obstruction	82	
intestinal regulator	20	
intestine; intestinal	134	
intradiscal pressure	148	
intravenous drip	21	
intravenous hyperalimentation (IVH)	21	
inversion	4	
involuntary movement	60	
inward circumduction	3	
iris	122	
iron deficiency	95	
ischemic cerebrovascular disease	65	
ischemic heart disease (IHD)	62	
ischium; ischial	132	
isometric contraction	59	
isotonic contraction	59	
itchiness	49	
itching	49	

J

Jacksonian seizure	59	
Janus kinase 3 defect	102	
jaundice	49	
jaw	114	
jejunum; jejunal	134	
jerk	52	
joint contracture	56	
jugular veins	118	
jumper's knee	56	
juvenile	49	

K

Kaposi sarcoma	76	

Kark amputation	18	
keratitis	71	
keratoconjunctivitis	71	
keratopathy	71	
Kernig sign	16	
ketoacidosis	93	
kidney	135	
kidney stone	86	
Klapp's creeping exercise	24	
Klenzack joint	28	
kneading	25	
knee	141	
knee disarticulation prosthesis	28	
knee joint	142	
knee orthosis (KO)	30	
knee-ankle-foot orthosis (KAFO)	30	
kneecap	142	
kneel sitting position	2	
kneeling position	2	
knock-knee	56	
knuckle bender	32	
Krukenberg amputation	18	
kwashiorkor	95	
kyphosis	54	

L

labor	89
labor paints	89
lacrimal gland	122
lacrimal sac	122
lacrimal bone	115
lacrimal passage obstruction	71
lactorrhea	92
lactose	153
lactose intolerance	95
ladder	33
lagophthalmos	71
language disorder	46
lap board	33
large intestine (bowel)	134
laryngeal cancer	73
laryngeal inlet	131
laryngeal polyp	73
laryngeal prominence	120
laryngeal reflex	151
laryngitis	73
larynx; laryngeal	131
Lasegue sign	16
late cerebellar cortical atrophy (LCCA)	65
latent errors	41
lateral bending	3
lateral femoral cutaneous nerve	145
lateral malleolus	141
lateral position	2
lateral pterygoid [muscle]	116
lateral rectus [muscle]	116
latissimus dorsi [muscle]	126
lavatory	33
laxative	20
lazy eye	70
learning disability	106
leather molded brace	29
leather works	23
left handed	149
leftward bending	3
leftward rotation	4
leg	141
leg discrepancy	5
lens	122
lesser trochanter	142
leukemia	97
leukemoid reaction	98
leukocyte	146
leukocytosis	98
leukoderma	76
leukopenia	98
leukorrhea	87
levator anguli oris [muscle]	116
levator ani [muscle]	133
levator scapulae [muscle]	139
levocardia	103
life style-related disease	95
life support	17
life therapy	22
lifestyle	17
lifting platform	33
light reflex	151
light sensation	147
lightheadedness	49
limbic system	120
line bisection test	8
linear fracture	54
lingua; lingual	123
lingual cancer	82
lipiduria	84
lissencephaly	103
liver	134
liver cancer	82
liver cell carcinoma	81
lobe	120
locomotion activity	5
long leg brace (LLB)	30
long opponens splint	31
long opponens wrist hand orthosis	29
long sitting position	2
long-standing	45
long-term care health facility	39
long-term care insurance facility	39
longissimus cervicis [muscle]	116
longissimus thoracis [muscle]	128
longitudinal ligaments	142
longus capitis [muscle]	116
longus colli [muscle]	116
loose abductor brace	30
loose stool	80
lordosis	54
Lorenz apparatus	29

Term	Page
low back pain	54
low blood pressure	63
low frequency current therapy	22
low grade fever	47
lower abdominal pain	82
lower back	125
lower extremity (limb)	141
—— amputation	18
—— varix	63
—— prosthesis for sport	28
lumbago	54
lumbar cord	126
lumbar nerve	126
lumbar orthosis	31
lumbar plexus	126
lumbar triangle	128
lumbosacral strain	55
lumbricals [muscle]	139
lump	49
lung	131
lung cancer	78
lung compliance	10
lung physiotherapy	21
lung volume	10
lupus erythematosus	90
luteinizing hormone	153
luxation	56
lying position	2
lymph node	129
—— tuberculosis	98
lymph vessel	129
lymphadenitis	98
lymphadenopathy	98
lymphangiectasis	98
lymphangiomyomatosis (LAM)	78
lymphangitis	98
lymphatic abnormality	98
lymphedema	98
lymphocele	99
lymphocyte	146
lymphohistiocytosis	99
lymphoma	99, 146
lymphopenia	49
lymphoproliferative syndrome	99
lymphosarcoma	99
lysosomal disease	93

M

Term	Page
macramé	23
macroglobulinemia	99
macrophage	146
macropsia	106
macrosomia	93
macula lutea (retinae)	122
macular degeneration	71
maculopathy	71
magnetic resonance angiography (MRA)	8
magnetic resonance imaging (MRI)	8
malabsorption syndrome	95
malformation syndrome	103
malignant	49
malleolar prosthesis	26, 28
malleolus; malleolar	141
malleus	115
malnutrition	95
malocculusion	82
malpractice	41
mammary gland	135
mandible; mandibular	114
mania	106
manic-depressive disorder (psychosis)	106
manual	136
manual braille writer	32
manual chest stretching	25
manual muscle testing (MMT)	8
maple syrup urine disease	103
marasmus	95
masculinization	93
massage	25
masseter [muscle]	116
masseter reflex	151
mastalgia	87
mastitis	87
mastoid process	115
mastoiditis	72
maternity	89
maxilla; maxillary	114
maxillary cancer	83
maximal voluntary ventilation (MVV)	10
measles	110
measurement of [body] weight	9
medial malleolus	141
medial otitis	73
medial pterygoid [muscle]	116
medial rectus [muscle]	116
median nerve	139
mediastinal tumor	78
medical interview	17
medical negligence	41
medical record review (audit)	41
medical rehabilitation	35
medical representative (MR)	41
medical social work	37
medical social worker (MSW)	36
medication	20
medicine	20
medulla oblongata	120
megacolon	82
megalencephaly	103
megasomia	93
melanoma	76
Ménière disease	67
meningioma	65
meningitis	65
meninx; meningeal	121
meniscus	142
menopausal syndrome	87

menopause	87	
menorrhagia	87	
menoxenia	87	
menstrual pain	87	
menstruation disturbance	87	
mental disorder	46	
mental retardation	106	
mental welfare center	38	
mentalis [muscle]	116	
mentum	114	
metabolic equivalents (METs, MET)	15	
metabolic rate	8	
metabolic syndrome	95	
metacarpal bone	137	
metacarpophalangeal (MP) joints	137	
metacarpus; metacarpal	136	
metal frame orthosis	29	
metatarsal arch	142	
metatarsal bar	30	
metatarsal bone	142	
metatarso-phalangeal (MTP) joints	142	
metatarsus; metatarsal	141	
method	15	
metrorrhagia	88	
micropsia	106	
microwave diathermy (therapy)	21	
miction pain	84	
micturition	149	
micturition desire	149	
micturition pain	84	
micturition reflex	151	
midbrain	121	
midcarpal joint	137	
middle constrictor [muscle] of pharynx	116	
middle ear	121	
middle nasal concha	115	
migraine	65	
mind-body therapy	22	
mini-mental state examination (MMSE)	12	
Minnesota Multiphasic Personality Inventory (MMPI)	12	
miosis	147	
misty vision	71	
mitral stenosis	62	
mitral valve	130	
mixed connective tissue disease	90	
mobility	60	
mobility impairment	60	
modular prosthesis	26, 28	
molar [tooth]	123	
monilethrix	103	
mononucleosis	99	
monoplegia	67	
mood disorder	106	
moon face	95	
motion	25, 60	
motor function test	8	
motor nerve	127	
motor root	129	
motor speech center	119	
mouth	123	
movement	25, 60	
moyamoya disease	67	
mucopolysaccharidosis	95	
mucosa; mucosal	49	
mucus; mucous	49	
multifidus [muscle]	126	
multiple health screening	7	
multiple pointing stick	32	
multiple sclerosis	69	
multiple system atrophy (MSA)	67	
multipurpose senior center	39	
mumps	109	
murmur	49	
muscle re-education exercise	23	
muscle relaxation exercise	23	
muscle strengthening exercise	23	
muscle weakness	58	
muscular atrophy	58	
muscular dystrophy	58	
muscular stiffness	58	
muscularis	134	
mustache	124	
mutism	106	
myasthenia	58	
myasthenia gravis	58	
myasthenic syndrome	58	
mycosis fungoides	99	
myelitis	67	
myelodysplastic syndrome (MDS)	99	
myelofibrosis	99	
myelography	8	
myeloma	99	
myelopathy	67	
myeloproliferative disorders (MPD)	99	
myocardial infarction	62	
myocardium; myocardial	130	
myoclonus	67	
myodesis	19	
myodesopsia	71	
myoelectric upper limb prosthesis	27	
myopia	71	
myotonic dystrophy	58	
myringitis	72	

N

nail	136
nape	114
narcolepsy	67
narcotics	20
naris	122
narrative-based medicine (NBM)	17
nasal cavity	122

Term	Page
nasal crest	115
nasal furuncle	73
nasal hemorrhage	73
nasal polyp	73
nasal reflex-neurosis	73
nasal septum	122
nasal vestibule	122
nasalis [muscle]	116
nasopharyngitis	73
national health insurance	37
nausea	49
navel	132
navicular	142
near reflex	151
near-miss or close-call incident	41
near-sightedness	71
neck	114
neck-shoulder-arm syndrome	56
necrosis	49
neonate; neonatal	50, 89
neoplasm	146
nephritis	84
nephrolith	86
nephropathy	84
nephrosclerosis	85
nephrosis	85
nephrotic syndrome	85
nerve conduction velocity (NCV)	8
nettle rush	77
neuralgia	67
neurapraxia	67
neuro-developmental [approach] to treatment	17
neurofibroma	67
neurofibromatosis	103
neurogenic bladder	85
neuropathic pain	50
neuropathy	67
neurophysiological approach	17
neurosis	106
neutral position	2
neutropenia	99
nevus	76
newborn	89
niacin	153
niacin deficiency	95
night blindness	70
night splint	31
night sweat	50
night terrors	106
nocturia	85
nocturnal amblyopia	70
nocturnal enuresis	44
nodular goiter	93
nonsteroidal antiinflammatory drugs (NSAIDs)	19
nontuberculous mycobacterial disease	110
noradrenaline	153
norepinephrine	153
norovirus	112
nose; nasal	122
nosebleed	73
nosocominal infection	110
nostril	122
numbness	50
nursery school	39
nutrition disorder	95
nyctalopia	70

O

Term	Page
obesity	95
objective audiometry	11
obsessive-compulsive disorder (OCD)	106
obstructive ventilator disturbance	78
obturator externus [muscle]	133
obturator internus [muscle]	133
obturator nerve	145
occipital bone	115
occipitalis [muscle]	116
occipitofrontalis [muscle]	116
occult blood	50
occupational disease	17
occupational therapist (OT)	35
occupational therapy	21
ocular dysmetria	11
ocular movement	147
ocular muscle	116
oculomotor nerve	117
oculus; ocular	122
odontobothritis	82
odynophagia	50
old-age home with moderate fee	39
old-sightedness	71
olecranon	136
olfactory bulb	123
olfactory disturbance	73
olfactory hyperesthesia	74
olfactory nerve	117
oligomenorrhea	88
oliguria	85
oliva; olivary body	121
olive-ponto-cerebellar atrophy (OPCA)	67
one leg test	8
oophoritis	88
open fracture	54
open reduction	19
operant behavior	12
ophthalmic artery	118
ophthalmometry	11
Oppenheimer splint	31
opponens digiti minimi [muscle]	139
opponens digiti minimi pedis [muscle]	144
opponens pollicis [muscle]	139
opposition	4

oppositional defiant disorder (ODD)	106	
oppressing feeling	50	
optic ataxia	71	
optic chiasma	121	
optic disc	122	
optic nerve	117	
optical winking reflex	151	
optometry	11	
oral aphtha	83	
oral cavity	123	
orbicularis oculi [muscle]	116	
——— reflex	151	
orbicularis oris [muscle]	116	
orbit; orbital	115	
orthophoria	147	
orthopnea	78	
orthoptist	35	
orthosis for scoliosis	31	
orthostatic hypotension	63	
oscitation	53	
ossification	58	
ossification of posterior longitudinal ligament (OPLL)	58	
osteitis	55	
osteitis deformans	55	
osteoarthritis	56	
osteoarthropathy	56	
osteogenesis imperfecta	55	
osteomalacia	55	
osteoporosis	55	
osteosarcoma	55	
osteosynthesis	19	
otalgia	72	
otitis externa	73	
otitis interna	73	
otitis media	73	
otodynia	72	
otosalpinx	121	
otosclerosis	73	
outcome	18	
outward circumduction	3	
ovarian cancer	88	
ovarian dysfunction	88	
ovary; ovarian	135	
overnutrition	95	
overtraining syndrome	55	
ovum; oval	135	
oxygen consumption	149	
oxygen dissociation curve	149	
oxygen uptake (intake)	10, 149	
oxyuriasis	109	

P

pain	50
pain disorder	106
pain killer	19
pain reliever	19
palate; palatine	123
palatine bone	115
palatine tonsil	123
palatine uvula	123
palm; palmar	136
palmar abduction	3
palmar adduction	3
palmar digital arteries	140
palmar flexion	4
palmar interossei [muscle]	139
palmaris brevis [muscle]	139
palmaris longus [muscle]	139
palpation	18
palpitation	50
palsy	67
pancreas; pancreatic	134
pancreatic cancer	82
pancreatitis	82
panic disorder	106
papillary muscle	130
papule	76
paraffin bath	25
paralysis	68
paranasal sinus	123
paraparesis	68

paraphasia	106
paraplegia	68
parasite	111
paraspinal muscle	126
parathyroid gland	114
parathyroid hormone (PTH)	153
paratyphoid fever	110
parenteral nutrition	20
paresis	68
paresthesia	68
parietal bone	115
Parkinson disease	65
parotiditis	73
partial bath	25
partial foot prosthesis	28
partial hand prosthesis	27
passive movement	25
past history	17
patella; patellar	142
patellar clonus	56
patellar tendon	142
——— reflex (PTR)	151
——— bearing (PTB) prosthesis	30
patellofemoral (PF) joint	142
pathological gambling	106
Pavlik harness	32
pectineus [muscle]	133
pectoralis major [muscle]	128
pectoralis minor [muscle]	128
pediculosis	110
pedophilia	106
peg board	23
pellagra	95
pelvis; pelvic	132
pemphigus	76
penis; penile	135
peptic ulcer	82
percent vital capacity	10
percussion	18

periarthritis scapulahumeralis	57	
perimetry	11	
periodontal disease	83	
peripheral neuropathy	67	
peritonitis	82	
permanent prosthesis	26	
perseverative tendency	50	
person with disabili-ties	36	
personality disorder	106	
perspiration	50	
pertussis	110	
pes	141	
phacomatosis	103	
phalanx [of foot]	142	
phalanx [of hand]	137	
phantom limb pain	50	
pharyngeal cancer	83	
pharyngeal reflex	151	
pharyngitis	74	
pharyngoconjunctival fever (PCF)	110	
pharynx; pharyngeal	131	
phenylketonuria	95	
pheochromocytoma	93	
phlebitis	63	
phlegm	51	
phobia	107	
phocomelia	103	
photoalgia	71	
photophobia	71	
photosensitivity	71	
physical dependence	46	
physical disability certificate	37	
physical medicine	35	
physical therapist (PT)	35	
physical therapy	21	
physiotherapy	21	
pica	107	
pigmentation	76	
pile	81	
pimple	76	
pinna	121
piriformis [muscle]	133
Pirogoff amputation	18
pisiform	137
piss	52
pituitary gland	120
placement ladder	33
placenta; placental	135
plantar	141
plantar fascia	144
plantar flexion	4
plantar interossei [muscle]	144
plantar muscle reflex	151
plantar reflex	151
plantaris [muscle]	144
plaque	50
plasma	146
plaster	34
plaster splint	34
plastic orthosis	29
platelet	146
platform crutch	32
pleural effusion	47
pleural mesothelioma	78
pleural plaque	50
pleurisy	78
pleuritis	78
plug fit type socket	26
plugged ear	73
pneumonia	79
pneumonoconiosis	79
pneumothorax	79
poisoning	50
polio[myelitis]	68
pollakiuria	85
pollenosis	74
polyangiitis	63
polyarteritis	63
polycystic kidney disease	85
polycythemia vera	100
polydactyly	103
polyendocrinopathy	93
polymyalgia rheumatica (PMR)	57
polymyositis	59
polymyositis / dermatomyosistis	59
polyp	50
polyphagia	107
polypnea	79
polyposia	50
polysaccharide	153
polyuria	85
pons	121
popliteal artery	145
popliteal fossa	141
popliteal lymph nodes	145
popliteal vein	145
popliteus [muscle]	144
portal hypertension	82
positron emission tomography (PET)	8
posterior cruciate ligament	142
posterior interosseous nerve	139
posterior longitudinal ligament	142
posterior meniscofemoral ligament	142
posterior standing position	2
postgastroectomy syndrome	82
posttraumatic stress disorder (PTSD)	107
postural drainage	25
postural exercise	24
postural supporting device	29
posture	2
postviral fatigue syndrome	68
potassium depletion	95
precocious puberty	93
pregnancy	89
prehension orthosis	30
premenstrual irregularity	87

premenstrual syndrome (PMS) 88
premolar [tooth] 123
presbyopia 71
prescription 18
pressure pill 19
prevocational occupational therapy 22
primary 50
primary nursing care requirement authorization 37
priority 41
private residential home 40
procerus [muscle] 116
proctaresia 101
progeria 103
prognosis; prognostic 18
projection 50
prolactin-producing adenoma 94
pronation 4
pronator quadratus [muscle] 139
pronator teres [muscle] 139
prone position 2
prostate gland; prostatic 135
prostatic abscess 85
prostatic cancer 85
prostatic hyperplasia 85
prostatic stone (calculus) 85
prostatism 85
prostatitis 85
prostatitis syndrome 85
prostatocystitis 85
prosthetic and orthotic treatment 21
prosthetic training 24
prosthetist and orthotist (PO) 35
protein 153
protein-energy malnutrition (PEM) 95
proteinuria 85
protocol 42
protozoan 111
protraction 4
protrusion 4
proximal interphalangeal (PIP) joints 137
proximal radioulnar joint 137
pruritus 49, 76
pseudohypoaldosteronism 94
pseudohypoparathyroidism 94
pseudolymphoma 146
psoas major [muscle] 126
psoas minor [muscle] 126
psoriasis 76
psychiatric rehabilitation 35
psychiatric social worker (PSW) 36
psychosis 107
psychosomatic disorder (PSD) 107
psychotropic 20
PTES transtibial prosthesis 30
pubic hair 124
pubis; pubic 132
public health center 40
pudendal nerve 133
pulmonary 131
pulmonary [viscous] resistance 10
pulmonary arteries 129
pulmonary edema 79
pulmonary embolism 79
pulmonary emphysema 78
pulmonary function 149
pulmonary rehabilitation 35
pulmonary thromboembolism 79
pulmonary trunk 129
pulmonary valve 129
pulpitis 83
PULSES Profile 15
pupil; pupillary 122
pupillary reflex 151
pure tone audiometry 11
purgative 20
purpura 76, 100
pursed lips breathing 24
push off 5
pyelonephritis 85
pylon prosthesis 28
pylorus; pyloric 134
pyonephrosis 85
pyramidal decussation 121
pyramidal process 115
pyramidal tract 121
—— disorder 68
pyrosis 48
pyuria 85

Q

quad cane 32
quadratus femoris [muscle] 144
quadratus lumborum [muscle] 133
quadriceps femoris [muscle] 144
quadrilateral socket 26
quadriplegia 68
quality assurance 42
quality of life (QOL) 15
questionnaire 15

R

rabies 110
rachitis 96
radial abduction 3
radial artery 140
radial deviation 3
radial flexion 4
radial fracture 54
radial nerve 139
radial vein 140
radiant heat therapy 22

Term	Page
radiating pain	50
radiotherapy	21
radioulnar triangular cartilage	137
radius; radial	137
rale	51
range of motion (ROM)	60
—— exercise	24
—— test (ROMT)	8
rapid eye movement (REM) sleep	148
—— behavior disorder	107
rash	75
reacher	33
reaction	150
rebound phenomenon	51
reciprocal walker	33
reciprocating gait orthosis (RGO)	30
reclining wheelchair	33
recommendations for lifestyle modification	17
recovery rehabilitation	35
recreation therapy	22
rectal cancer	82
rectum; rectal	134
rectus abdominis [muscle]	133
rectus femoris [muscle]	144
recumbent position	2
red blood cell (RBC)	146
reduction	19
reevaluation	15
reflex	150
refraction test	11
refractometry	11
regular checkup	7
rehabilitation	35
rehabilitation counseling	37
rehabilitation doctor	36
rehabilitation engineering	35
rehabilitation facilities for the visually impaired persons	40
rehabilitation service	37
relative metabolic rate (RMR)	8
relaxation	51
remedy	20
remission	18, 51
renal	135
renal amyloidosis	85
renal artery	133
renal calculus	86
renal carcinoma	85
renal failure	85
renal infarction	86
renal ischemia	86
renal osteodystrophy	96
renal tubular acidosis	86
renal tubular dysfunction	86
repetitive saliva swallowing test (RSST)	8
residual function	15
residual hearing	73
residual urine	86
residual volume	10
resistance (resistive) exercise	25
resistance to thyroid hormone	94
respiration; respiratory	24, 149
respiratory center	119
respiratory failure	79
respiratory function	149
respiratory muscle	128
respiratory paralysis	79
respiratory quotient	149
respiratory resistance	10
respiratory sound	149
respiratory tract	131
response	152
restroom	33
retching reflex	152
retina; retinal	122
retinal artery	118
retinal vein	118
retinopathy	71
retraction	4
retrusion	4
Rett syndrome	107
reverse knuckle bender	32
rheumatic fever	110
rheumatism	56
rheumatoid arthritis	57
rhinitis	74
rhinopolypus	73
rhinorrhea	51
rhomboid major [muscle]	126
rhomboid minor [muscle]	126
rhonchus	51
rib	128
rickets	96
rickettsia	111
Riemenbugel (RB)	32
right handed	149
rightward bending	3
rightward rotation	4
rigid orthosis	29
rigidity	51
risk management	42
risorius [muscle]	116
roam	53
rod exercise	24
rod klenzack	29
Rorschach Test	12
rose spot	76
rotation	4
rotator cuff	137
rotatores [muscle]	126
rubbing	25
rubella	110
rubeola	110
rubor	75
rupture	59
rupture of membranes	89
Rye syndrome	65

S

Term	Page
saccharometabolic disorder	96

sacral nerve	127	
sacral plexus	127	
sacroiliac orthosis	31	
sacrospinalis [muscle]	126	
sacrum; sacral	125	
sadomasochism	107	
safety knee	32	
salivary gland	123	
—— atrophy	83	
—— tumor	83	
salmonella	111	
salpingitis	88	
sanatorium type sickbed	38	
sanatorium type ward	38	
sanding	23	
sandplay therapy	22	
saphenous nerve	145	
saphenous vein	145	
SAPHO syndrome	57	
sarcoidosis	90	
sarcoma	146	
satisfaction in daily life (SDL)	15	
sausage-like fingers	51	
savant syndrome	107	
scabies	76	
scale	15	
scalenus anterior muscle	116	
scalp	124	
scalp hair	124	
scaphoid [bone]	137	
scapula	128	
scapulohumeral periarthritis	57	
scar	51	
scarlet fever	110	
schizoaffective disorder	108	
schizophrenia	108	
schizophreniform disorder	108	
schizotypal disorder	108	
school for the deaf	40	
sciatic	132	
sciatic nerve	133	

sciatic neuralgia 68
sciatica 68
scissors gait 60
sclera; scleral 122
scleroderma 76
sclerosis 51, 68
scoliosis 55
scorbutus 96
score 16
scotoma 122
scrotum; scrotal 135
scurvy 96
secondary 51
sedative 20
seizure 44, 45
self-help device 33
sella turcica 115
semen 135
semi-sitting position 2
semicircular canals 121
semicoma 51
senile 51
sensory center 119
sensory integrative therapy (approach) 22
sensory speech center 119
sepsis 110
septal deviation 74
septum; septal 130
seronegative spondyloarthropathy 90
serosa; serous 134
serratus anterior [muscle] 129
serratus posterior inferior [muscle] 126
serratus posterior superior [muscle] 126
serum 146
sesamoid bone [of foot] 143
sesamoid bone [of hand] 137
severe acute respira-tory syndrome (SARS) 79
severe pain 50

sexual deviation 108
sexually transmitted diseases (STD) 88
shared psychotic disorder 108
sheltered workshop 40
shin 141
shingles 110
shoe horn brace (SHB) 30
shoe orthosis 30
short leg brace (SLB) 30
short opponens hand orthosis 30
short opponens splint 31
short stature 94
short stay 37
shoulder 136
shoulder blade 128
shoulder disarticulation prosthesis 27
shoulder joint 28, 137
shoulder orthosis 30
shoulder-hand syndrome 55
shuffle alternate gait 60
shuffle simultaneous gait 60
side-lying position 2
sign 16
Silesian band 32
silicon rubber prosthesis 27
simian hand 69
simple fracture 54
Simple Motor Test for Cerebral Palsy (SMTCP) 8
Simple Test for Evaluating Hand Function (STEF) 9
simultanagnosia 65
single axis knee 29
single parent support facility 40
single photon emission computed tomography (SPECT) 9
sinistrocardia 103
sinistromanual 149
sinusitis 74

Term	Page
sitting position	2
—— on the bed	2
skin	124
skull	115
sleep	148
sleep apnea syndrome (SAS)	79
sleep architecture	148
sleep cycle	148
sleep[ing] disorder	46, 108
sleep efficiency	148
sleep onset	148
sleep stage	148
sleeping pill	20
sleeplessness	108
slim disease	96
small intestine (bowel)	134
smallpox	110
snap	52
sneezing	51
snore	51
social history	17
social hospitalization	37
social insurance office	40
social rehabilitation	35
social skill training (SST)	24
social welfare office	40
social work	37
social worker	36
soft dressing	32
soft orthosis	29
sole	141
soleus [muscle]	144
solid ankle cushion heel (SACH) foot	28
somatization disorder	108
somatoform disorder	108
somatosensory evoked potentials	9
somnolence	51
sore	51
sore throat	51
spasm	51
spasticity	51
spatial visual acuity	148
special elderly nursing home	40
special functioning hospital	38
speech audiogram	11
speech audiometry	11
speech center	119
speech discrimination score	11
speech disorder (im-pediment)	66
speech language hearing therapist (ST)	36
speech reception threshold	11
sperm	135
spermatic cord tortion	88
spermatocele	88
sphenoid [bone]	115
sphenoidal sinus	123
sphygmomanometry	9
spina bifida	103
spinal canal	125
spinal cord	127
—— disease (SCD)	69
—— injury (SCI)	69
spinal deformity	57
spinal ganglion	127
spinal motor neuron	148
spinal muscular atrophy	58
spinal nerve	127
spinal progressive muscular atrophy	58
spinal reflex	151
spinal segment	127
spinal [canal] stenosis	55
spinalis cervicis [muscle]	126
spinalis thoracis [muscle]	126
spine; spinal	125
spinobulbospinal reflex	151
spirometer	10
spleen; splenic	146
splenic artery	133
splenic vein	133
splenius capitis [muscle]	126
splenius cervicis [muscle]	126
spondylitis	55
spondylitis deformans	55
spondylolisthesis	55
spondylolysis	55
spondylosis	55
spoon nail	51
sprain	57
sputum	51
squint	71
[walking] stick	32
stabilizer	29
stage	16
staggering walk	6
stair climbing	5
stairlift	34
stammering	52
stamping	23
Standard Language Test of Aphasia (SLTA)	9
standing	5
standing on one leg	5
standing on tiptoe	5
standing position	2
stapes	115
Staphylococcus aureus	111
staphylococcus; staphylococcal	111
stenosing tenosynovitis	59
stenosis	51
step	5
step length	5
step width	5
steppage gait	60
stepping reflex	152
stereognosis	52
sterility	89
sternoclavicular joint	128
sternocleidomastoid [muscle]	129
sternocostal joint	128

sternum; sternal 128	subtalar joint 143	symmetrical tonic neck
sternutaion 51	suction type above knee	reflex 152
stiff neck and shoulder 59	prosthesis 29	sympathetic trunk 121
stiff skin 76	suction type socket 26	symptom 52
stoma 32	sudden cardiac death (SCD) 62	syncope 47, 52
stomach 134	sunburn 52	syphilis 110
stomach cancer 81	suntan 52	syringe 21
stomatitis 82	superficial palmar arch 140	syringomyelia 69
strabismus 71	superficial peroneal	systemic bone disease 55
straight leg raising (SLR)	(fibular) nerve 145	**T**
test 9	superior gemellus [muscle]	
strained back 55	144	T cane 32
strawberry tongue 52	superior gluteal nerve 145	tachycardia 62
Streptococcus pneumoniae 111	superior pharyngeal	tachypnea 79
streptococcus; strepto-	constrictor [muscle] 116	tactile materials for the
coccal 111	supination 4	floor 34
stress fracture 54	supinator [muscle] 139	talar tilt 143
stretching exercise 25	supine position 2	talipes 57
stride 6	supportive occupational	talocalcaneonavicular joint
stride length 6	therapy 21	143
stride width 6	supraorbital nerve 117	talocrural joint 143
stroke 66	supraspinatus [muscle] 139	talus; talar 143
stroking 25	sural nerve 145	tardive 52
stump pain 50	surface heating therapy 22	tarry stool 82
stump training 24	surgical history 17	tarsal [bones] 143
stupor 52	suspended animation 52	tarsal tunnel syndrome
stuttering 52	susurrus aurium 72	(TTS) 69
sty 71	swallowing 148	tarsometatarsal joints 143
styloid process 137	swallowing center 119	tarsus; tarsal 141
subacromial bursa 137	swallowing function 148	taste 148
subarachnoid space 121	swallowing grade 16	temple; temporal 114
subarachnoidal	swallowing reflex 152	temporal bone 115
hemorrhage (SAH) 66	swallowing training 24	temporalis [muscle] 116
subclavian artery 129	sweat gland 124	temporary lower limb
subclavian vein 129	sweating 50	prosthesis 28
subclavius [muscle] 139	swelling 47	temporary prosthesis 26
subcutaneous hemorrhage	swing-through gait 60	temporary upper limb
(bleeding) 48	swing-to gait 60	prosthesis 27
subdural hematoma 66	swinging flashing test 11	temporomandibular
subdural hemorrhage 66	Swiss lock knee joint 33	disorders (TMD) 57
subdural space 121	swollen tonsils 52	temporoparietalis [muscle] 116
subluxation 57	Syme amputation 18	tenderness 52
subscapularis [muscle] 139	Syme prosthesis 29	tendinous cords 130

tendon grafting	19	thorough medical checkup	7	tonometry	11
tendon reflex	152	three-point gait	60	tonsillitis	74
tendon transfer	19	threshold	16	tooth	123
tendonitis	59	throat	131	Toronto hip abduction orthosis	29
tendovaginitis	59	thrombocythemia	100	torsion dystonia	58
tennis elbow	57	thrombocytopenia	100	torticollis	55
tenosynovitis	59	thrombolytic	20	total lung capacity (TLC)	10
tensor fasciae latae [muscle]	144	thrombophlebitits	63	Tower of Hanoi	13
teres major [muscle]	139	thrombus	52	toxic shock syndrome (TSS)	110
teres minor [muscle]	139	thumb	136	toxoplasma	111
terminal care	35	thumb localizing test	9	toxoplasmosis	110
terminal device	28	thymus [gland]	128	trachea: tracheal	131
terminal nerve	117	thymus hyperplasia	100	tracheal bifurcation	131
test of activities of daily living	9	thyroid gland	114	tracheal cartilage	131
testicle; testicular	135	thyroid nodule	93	trachoma	110
testicular tumor	88	thyroid tumor	94	traction therapy	22
testis	135	thyroid-stimulating hormone (TSH)	153	training	24
tetanus	110	thyroid-stimulating hormone receptor disease	94	training in parallel bar	24
thalamic hand	52			tranquilizer	20
thalamus; thalamic	121			trans-humeral prosthesis	27
Thematic Apperception Test (TAT)	13	thyroiditis	94	trans-radial prosthesis	27
thenar muscle	139	thyrotropin	153	trans-tibial prosthesis	28
therapeutic electrical stimulation (TES)	21	thyrotropin-releasing hormone (TRH)	153	transcutaneous electrical nerve stimulation (TENS)	21
therapeutic eye exercises	11	tibia; tibial	143	transfer activity	5
therapeutic orthosis	29	tibial nerve	145	transient	52
therapy	22	tibialis anterior [muscle]	144	transient ischemic attack (TIA)	66
therapy program	18	tibialis posterior [muscle]	144	transitive motion	25
thermotherapy	22	tidal volume	10	transparency	42
thiamin deficiency	96	tilt table	34	transplant	19
thigh	141	Timed Up and Go (TUG) test	9	transplantation	19
thigh bone	142			transverse process	125
Thomas splint	31	tinea pedis	76	transverse retinacular ligament	137
Thomas weight bearing orthosis	30	Tinel sign	16		
		tinnitus	72	transverse tarsal joint	143
thoracic	128	toe	141	transversus abdominis [muscle]	133
thoracic cavity	128	toe loop	33		
thoracic duct	129	toe prosthesis	28	trapezium	137
thoracic nerve	129	toe reflex	152	trapezius [muscle]	126
thoracic orthosis	31	toileting	5	trapezoid	137
thorax	128	tongue	123		
		tongue cancer	82		

traumatic brain injury (TBI) 66	ulnar vein 140	urolithiasis 86
traumatic cervical syndrome 55	ultra-low temperature therapy 22	urticaria 77
treadmill test (TMT) 9	ultrasonography 9	uterine myoma 88
treatment 22	ultraviolet therapy 22	uterine rupture 88
tremor 66	umbilical artery 133	uterine sarcoma 88
triceps [muscle] of calf 144	umbilical cord 135	uterine tube 135
triceps branchii [muscle] 139	umbilical vein 133	uterus; uterine 135
triceps reflex 152	umbilicus; umbilical 132	uveitis 71

V

trichomoniasis 110	undernutrition 52	vaccination 22
trigeminal nerve 117	unilateral lobar emphysema 79	vaccine 22
triplegia 69	unit [joint] 26	vagina; vaginal 135
tripped cane 32	upper arm 136	vaginal discharge 87
triquetrum 137	upper extremity (limb) 136	vagus nerve 117
trisomy 13 syndrome 103	── amputation 18	valve 130
trisomy 18 syndrome 102	upright position 3	valvular heart disease 62
trochlear nerve 117	uremia 86	varicella 111
tubal obstruction 73	ureter; ureteral 135	varix 63
tubal stenosis 73	ureterolithiasis 86	vas deferens 135
tuberculosis 79	urethra; urethral 135	vascular murmur 63
tubular necrosis 86	urethral sphincter 133	vasculitis syndrome 63
tummy 132	urethral stenosis 86	vasodilator drug 20
tumor 146	urethral stricture 86	vasopressin 153
tuning fork 11	urethral syndrome 86	vasovagal syndrome 69
twist 52	urethritis 86	vastus intermedius [muscle] 144
two and one point gait 60	urethrostenosis 86	vastus lateralis [muscle] 144
two-point discrimination 13	urethrovaginal sphincter 133	vastus medialis [muscle] 144
two-steps breathing 24	uric acid 153	vaulting gait 60
tympanic membrane 121	── metabolic disorder 96	vegetative dystonia 69
typhoid fever 110	urinal 34	vein; venous 129
typhus 111	urinary calculus 86	velar sound 52
	urinary disturbance 86	velocardiofacial syndrome 103

U

	urinary incontinence 86	vena cava 130
ulcer 52	urinary tract candidiasis 86	ventilation threshold 10
ulcerative colitis 80	urinary tract infection (UTI) 86	ventricle; ventricular 130
ulna; ulnar 137	urinary tract stone disease 86	ventricular septal defect (VSD) 62
ulnar adduction 3	urinary tubule 135	venule 130
ulnar artery 140	urinate 52	verruca 77
ulnar deviation 3	urination 149	vertebra prominens 115
ulnar flexion 4	urine diverters 34	vertebra; vertebral 125
ulnar nerve 139	urine; uric; urinary 149	vertebral artery 118
ulnar tunnel syndrome 57	urolith 86	vertebral canal 125

vertebral column	125
vertebral-spinal cord tumor	55
vertical suspension test	9
vertigo	52
vessel	130
vestibular aqueduct	118
vestibular nerve	117
vestibular postural reflex	152
vestibular reflex	152
vestibular sense	148
vestibulocochlear nerve	117
vestibulospinal reflex	152
videoendoscopy	9
videofluorography	9
virilism	94
virus; viral	111
visceral inversion	102
visceral nerve	133
visceromotor nerve	133
viscerosensory nerve	133
visiting nursing	37
visiting rehabilitation	37
visual acuity	148
—— correction inspection	11
visual angle	148
visual distortion	71
visual feedback	148
visual filed defect	72
visual field test	11
visual hallucination	105
visual impairment	72
visual recognition memory test	11
visual sense (sensation)	148
vital capacity	10
vitamin	153
vitamin A deficiency	96
vitamin C deficiency	96
vitamin D deficiency	94
vitiligo	77
vitreous body	122
vocal cord	131
—— palsy	74
—— paralysis	74
vocal fold	131
vocal nodule	74
vocational facility	40
vocational rehabilitation	35
vocational training	24
voice box	131
voiding	149
volitional (voluntary) movement	25
vomiting	52
vomiting reflex	152
von Rosen apparatus (splint)	31

W

waddling gait	60
walk[ing]	6
walk with support	6
walk without help	6
walker	33
walking rate	5
walking support	32
wand	32
wander	53
ward	38
wart	77
weakness	53
Wegener's granulomatosis	90
weight loss	53
[body] weight	9
weight reduction	53
welfare center for the elderly	40
Wernicke center (area)	119
Western Aphasia Battery [Test]	9
wheelchair	33
wheelchair activity	5
wheezes	53
whiskers	124
white blood cell (WBC)	146
white matter	121
whooping cough	110
Williams type lumbosacral orthosis	31
windpipe	131
wink reflex	151
Wisconsin Card Sorting Test	9
wisdom tooth	123
womb	135
wood carving	23
woodwork[ing]	23
work arm	27
work tolerance	9
wrist	136
wrist disarticulation prosthesis	27
wrist joint	28, 137
wrong-site surgery	42
wryneck	55

X, Y, Z

xeroderma	77
xiphisternum	128
xiphoid process	128
XO syndrome	103
yawn	53
yellow spot	122
zona	110
zygomatic bone	115
zygomatic nerve	117
zygomaticus major [muscle]	117
zygomaticus minor [muscle]	117

Abbreviations
(略語一覧)

A

ADHD	attention-deficit/hyperactivity disorder 注意欠陥/多動性障害	
ADL	activities of daily living　日常生活動作	
AE amputation	above elbow amputation　上肢(AE)切断	
AED	automated external defibrillator　自動体外式除細動器	
AFO	ankle foot orthosis　短下肢装具	
AK amputation	above knee amputation　大腿(AK)切断	
AKA	arthrokinematic approach　関節運動学的アプローチ	
ALS	amyotrophic lateral sclerosis　筋萎縮性側索硬化症	
AN	anorexia nervosa　神経性食思不振症	
AP	angina pectoris　狭心症	
APDL	activities parallel to daily living　生活関連動作	
ARP	alcohol rehabilitation program　アルコール中毒リハプログラム	
AS	ankylosing spondylitis　強直性脊椎炎	
ASD	acute stress disorder　急性ストレス障害	
ASO	arteriosclerosis obliterans　閉塞性動脈硬化〔症〕	
ATNR	asymmetric tonic neck reflex　非対称性緊張性頸反射	
ATR	Achilles tendon reflex　アキレス腱反射	

B

BADL	basic activities of daily living　基本日常生活動作	
BADS	Behavioural Assessment of the Dysexecutive Syndrome 遂行機能障害症候群の行動評価	
BDI	Beck depression index　ベックうつ病自己評価尺度	
BE amputation	below elbow amputation　上腕(BE)切断	
BFO	balanced forearm orthosis　平均前腕装具	
BGT	Bender Gestalt test　ベンダーゲシュタルト検査	
BI	Barthel Index　バーセルインデックス	
BIT	behavioural inattention test　行動無視検査	
BK amputation	below knee amputation　下腿(BK)切断	
BMI	body mass index　体格指数	
BMR	basal metabolic rate　基礎代謝率	
BN	bulimia nervosa　神経性大食症	
BP	blood pressure　血圧	
Brs stage	Brunnstrom stage　ブルンストロームステージ	

C

CAD	coronary artery disease	冠[状]動脈[性心]疾患
CC	chief complaint	主訴
CCM; COCM	congestive cardiomyopathy	うっ血型心筋症
CD	conduct disorder	行為障害
CDH	congenital dislocation of hipjoint	先天性股関節脱臼
CDT	Clock Drawing Test	時計描画テスト
CHART	Craig handicap assessment and reporting technique クレイグ・ハンディキャップ評価・報告法	
CHD	coronary heart disease	冠[状]動脈[性]心疾患
CHF	congestive heart failure	うっ血性心不全
CM	cardiomyopathy	心筋症
CM joint	carpometacarpal joint	手根中手関節
CMR	congenital muscular dystrophy	先天性筋ジストロフィー
CN	cranial nerves	脳神経
COPD	chronic obstructive pulmonary disease	慢性閉塞性肺疾患
Cord-T	co-ordination test	協調性テスト
CP	cerebral [infantile] palsy	脳性[小児]麻痺
CPM therapy	continuative passive motion therapy	持続的他動運動療法
CPR	cardiopulmonary resuscitation	心肺蘇生法
CQI	continuous quality improvement	継続的質の向上,改善
CT	computed tomography	コンピュータ断層撮影診断[法]
CVA	cerebrovascular accident (stroke)	脳血管障害(広義の脳卒中)
CVD	cerebrovascular disease (disorder)	脳血管疾患(障害)

D

DAM intelligence test	draw-a-man intelligence test	人物画知能検査
DCM	dilated cardiomyopathy	拡張型心筋症
DD	developmental disability/disorder	発達障害
DH	drug history	薬歴
DIP joint	distal interphalangeal joint	遠位指(趾)節間関節
DMD	Duchenne muscular dystrophy	デュシェーヌ型ジストロフィ
DQ	development quotient	発達指数
DR	diabetic retinopathy	糖尿病[性]網膜症
DTVP	developmental test of visual perception	視覚発達検査

E

EALD	extended activities of daily living	拡大ADL
EBM	evidence-based medicine	証拠に基づいた医療
ECG	electrocardiogram; electrocardiography	心電図;心電図検査[法]
EDS	Ehlers-Danlos syndrome	エーラース・ダンロス症候群

EEG	electroencephalogram; electroencephalography 脳波；脳波検査〔法〕	
EMG	electromyogram; electromyography　筋電図；筋電図検査〔法〕	
EPF	Employees' Pension Fund　厚生年金制度	
ESRD	end-stage renal disease　末期腎疾患	

F

FH	family history　家族歴	
FIM	functional independence measure　機能的自立度評価法	
Frx	fracture　骨折	

G

GAD	generalized anxiety disorder　全般性不安障害	
GBS	Guillain-Barré syndrome　ギラン(ギヤン)−バレー症候群	
GCS	Glasgow coma scale　グラスゴー昏睡尺度	
GH	growth hormone　成長ホルモン	
GID	gender identity disorder　性同一性障害	
GMFCS	gross motor function classification system 粗大運動機能分類システム	

H

HDS-R	Hasegawa dementia scale, revised 長谷川式簡易認知症評価スケール改訂版	
HIV	human immunodeficiency virus　ヒト免疫不全ウイルス	
HKAFO	hip-knee-ankle-foot orthosis　骨盤帯付き長下肢装具	
HPI	history of present illness　現病歴	
HR	heart rate　心拍数	
HTP	house-tree-person test　家屋−樹木−人物画法テスト	

I

ICD	International Statistical Classification of Diseases and Related Health Problems　疾病および関連保健問題の国際統計分類	
ICEROSS	Icelandic roll-on silicone socket　シリコン製内ソケット	
ICF	International Classification of Functioning, Disability and Health 国際生活機能分類	
ICIDH	International Classification of Impairments, Disabilities and Handicaps　国際障害分類	
IDDM	insulin-dependent diabetes mellitus　インスリン依存性糖尿病	
Ig	immunoglobulin　免疫グロブリン	
IQ	intelligent quotient　知能指数	
ISNCSCI	International Standards for Neurological Classification of Spinal Cord Injury　脊髄損傷後の残存自律神経機能の国際評価基準	

ISO	International Organization for Standardization	国際標準化機構
ISS	intelligent standard score	知能偏差値
ITP	idiopathic thrombocytopenic purpura 特発性血小板減少性紫斑病	
ITPA	Illinois Test of Psycholinguistic Abilities イリノイ精神言語能力検査	
IVH	intravenous hyperalimentation	経静脈高カロリー輸液

J

JCS	Japan coma scale	日本式昏睡尺度
JDDST-R	Denver Developmental Screening Test, revised Japanese version　改訂日本版デンバー式発達スクリーニング検査	
JOA score	The Japanese Orthopaedic Association score 日本整形外科学会股関節機能判定基準	
JRA	juvenile rheumatoid arthritis	若年性関節リウマチ
JSS-H	The Japan stroke scale — higher cortical function 脳卒中高次脳機能障害重症度スケール	
JSS-M	The Japan stroke scale — mortality 脳卒中運動機能障害重症度スケール	

K

K-ABC	Kaufman Assessment Battery for Children カウフマン児童知能検査	
KAFO	knee-ankle-foot orthosis	長下肢装具
KO	knee orthosis	膝装具

L

LASMI	Life Assessment Scale for the Mentally Ill 精神障害者社会生活評価尺度	
LCCA	late cerebellar cortical atrophy	晩発性小脳皮質萎縮症
LD	learning disability	学習障害
LLB	long leg brace	長下肢装具

M

MASA	The Mann Assessment of Swallowing Ability マン嚥下機能評価尺度	
MDS	myelodysplastic syndrome	骨髄異形成症候群
MG	myasthenia gravis	重症筋無力症
MH	marital history	結婚歴
MI	myocardial infarction	心筋梗塞〔症〕
MMPI	Minnesota multiphasic personality inventory ミネソタ多面人格目録	

MMSE	mini-mental state examination	簡易知能検査
MMT	manual muscle testing	徒手筋力検査法
MP joint	metacarpophalangeal joint	中手指節関節
MPD	myeloproliferative disorders	骨髄増殖疾患群
MR	mental retardation	精神遅滞
MRA	magnetic resonance angiography	磁気共鳴血管造影〔法〕
MRA	malignant rheumatoid arthritis	悪性関節リウマチ
MRI	magnetic resonance imaging	磁気共鳴画像〔法〕
MS	multiple sclerosis	多発性硬化症
MSW	medical social worker	医療ソーシャルワーカー
MTP joint	metatarso-phalangeal	中足趾節関節

N

NBM	narrative-based medicine	物語に基づいた医療
NCV	nerve conduction velocity	神経伝道速度
NGO	non-governmental organization	非政府組織
NPO	non-profit (not-for-profit) organization	非営利組織

O

OA	osteoarthritis	変形性関節症
OCD	obsessive-compulsive disorder	強迫性障害
ODA	official development assistance	政府開発援助
ODD	oppositional defiant disorder	反抗挑戦性障害
OP	osteoporosis	骨粗鬆(しょう)症
OPCA	olive-ponto-cerebellar atrophy	オリーブ橋小脳萎縮症
OPLL	ossification of posterior longitudinal ligament	後縦靱帯骨化症
OT	occupational therapist	作業療法士

P

PANSS scale	positive and negative syndrome scale	陽性・陰性症状評価尺度
PD	panic disorder	パニック障害
PDD	pervasive developmental disorder	広汎〔性〕発達障害
PEM	protein-energy malnutrition	蛋白質エネルギー栄養障害
PET	positron emission tomography	陽電子放出断層撮影〔法〕
PF joint	patellofemoral joint	膝蓋大腿関節
PH	past history	既往歴
PI	present illness	現病
PIP joint	proximal interphalangeal joint	近位指節間関節
PLMD	periodic limb movement disorder	周期性四肢運動障害
PM/DM	polymyositis/dermatomyositis	多発〔性〕筋炎/皮膚筋炎
PMD	progressive muscular dystrophy	進行性筋ジストロフィー

PMR	polymyalgia rheumatica	リウマチ性多〔発性〕筋痛症
PN	polyarteritis nodosa	結節性多発〔性〕動脈炎
PNF technique	proprioceptive neuro-muscular facilitation technique 固有受容性神経筋促進法	
PO	prosthetist and orthotist	義肢・装具士
PSD	psychosomatic disorder	心身症
PSW	psychiatric social worker	精神保健福祉士
PT	physical therapist	理学療法士
PTB	patellar tendon-bearing	膝蓋腱加重式
PTEG	percutaneous trans-esophageal gastrotubing (gastrostomy) 経皮経食道胃管ドレナージ	
PTES	prothèse tibiale à emboîtage supracondylien transtibial prosthesis　PTES式下腿義足	
PTR	patellar tendon reflex	膝蓋腱反射
PTSD	posttraumatic stress disorder	心的外傷後ストレス障害
PULSES profile	physical condition, upper limb function, lower limb function, sensory function, excretory function, support profile　身体状況, 上肢機能, 下肢機能, 感覚機能, 排尿・排泄機能プロフィール	

Q, R

QOL	quality of life	〔日常〕生活の質
RA	rheumatoid arthritis	関節リウマチ
RCM	restrictive cardiomyopathy	拘束型心筋症
REHAB	rehabilitation	リハビリテーション
RF	rheumatoid factor	リウマトイド因子
RGO	reciprocating gait orthosis	交互歩行装具
RMR	relative metabolic rate	エネルギー代謝率
ROM	range of motion	関節可動域
ROMT	range of motion test	関節可動域テスト
RSD	reflex sympathetic dystrophy	反射性交感神経性ジストロフィー
RSST	repetitive saliva swallowing test	反復唾液嚥下テスト
RV	residual volume	残気量

S

SACH foot	solid ankle cushion heel foot	サッチ足部
SAH	subarachnoidal hemorrhage	くも膜下出血
SAPHO syndrome	synovitis-acne-pustulosis-hyperostosis osteomyelitis syndrome　SAPHO(滑膜-痤瘡-囊胞症-骨化過剰骨髄炎)症候群	
SARS	severe acute respiratory syndrome	重症急性呼吸器症候群
SCD	spinal cord disease	脊髄疾患

SCD	spinal cord disease	脊髄疾患
SCI	spinal cord injury	脊髄損傷
SCSIT	Southern California sensory integration tests 南カリフォルニア感覚統合検査	
SDL	satisfaction in daily life	日常生活満足度
SDS	self-rating depression scale	自己評価抑うつ尺度
SF-36	medical outcomes study short form-36 health survey SF-36健康調査	
SGRQ	St George's respiratory questionnaire	聖ジョージ〔病院〕呼吸障害質問票
SH	social history	社会歴
SHB	shoe horn brace	靴べら式装具
SIAS	stroke impairment assessment set	脳卒中機能障害評価法
SLB	short leg brace	短下肢装具
SLR test	straight leg raising test	下肢伸展挙上試験
SLTA	standard language test of aphasia	標準失語症検査
SMTCP	simple motor test for cerebral palsy	脳性麻痺簡易運動検査
SOM	serious otitis media	滲出性中耳炎
SPECT	single photon emission computed tomography 単一陽電子断層撮影〔法〕	
SR	systems review	病歴要約,系統別再調査
SST	social skill training	社会生活技能訓練
ST	speech language hearing therapist	言語聴覚士
STEF	Simple Test for Evaluating Hand Function	簡易上肢機能テスト
SUBI	subjective well-being inventory	心の健康自己評価質問紙

T

TAT	thematic apperception test	主題統覚検査
TB	tuberculosis	結核
TBI	traumatic brain injury	脳外傷,外傷性脳損傷
TENS	transcutaneous electrical nerve stimulation	経皮的電気刺激〔法〕
TES	therapeutic electrical stimulation	治療的電気刺激〔法〕
TMD	temporomandibular disorders	顎関節症
TMT	treadmill test	トレッドミル試験
TTS	tarsal tunnel syndrome	足根管症候群

U, V

US	ultrasonography	超音波検査〔法〕
UTI	urinary tract infection	尿路感染症
VC	vital capacity	肺活量
VE	videoendoscopy	ビデオ内視鏡検査〔法〕
VF	video fluorography	ビデオ(X線)造影検査検査〔法〕

W

WAB; WABT　Western aphasia battery [test]　ウェスタン失語症統合検査
WAIS-R　Wechsler adult intelligence scale, revised
　　　　　　ウェクスラー成人知能検査〔評価尺度〕改訂版
WCST　　Wisconsin card sorting test　ウィスコンシンカード分類検査
WMS-R　Wechsler memory scale, revised
　　　　　　ウェクスラー記憶検査〔評価尺度〕改訂版
WPPSI-R　Wechsler preschool and primary scale of intelligence, revised　ウェクスラー就学前・小学生知能検査〔評価尺度〕改訂版

Y, Z

Y-G test　Yatabe-Guilford test　矢田部・ギルフォード性格検査，Y-G テスト
ZKS　　　Zentrale Koordinationsstörung syndrome　中枢性協調障害

【著者紹介】

清水雅子(しみず・まさこ)
金沢市生まれ
岡山大学大学院教育学研究科 英語教育専攻修士課程修了
元・川崎医療福祉大学医療福祉学部/大学院医療福祉学研究科 教授

服部しのぶ(はっとり・しのぶ)
名古屋市生まれ
オーストラリア・クイーンズランド州ボンド大学大学院(応用言語学TESOL専攻)修了
現在,藤田保健衛生大学医療科学部准教授

参考文献

- 寺澤芳雄:英語語源辞典.研究社,1997.
- 日本リハビリテーション医学会(編):リハビリテーション医学用語集 第7版.文光堂,2007.
- 高久史麿(総監修),ステッドマン医学大辞典編集委員会(編):ステッドマン医学大辞典 改訂第6版.メジカルビュー社,2008.
- 長崎重信(編):見て学ぶ作業療法の極意 イラスト作業療法 ブラウン・ノート:850のイラストで極める.メジカルビュー社,2008.
- 伊藤正男,井村裕夫,高久史麿(編):医学書院医学大辞典 第2版.医学書院,2009.
- 野村 嶬(編),奈良 勲,鎌倉矩子(シリーズ監修):標準理学療法学・作業療法学 基礎分野 解剖学 第3版.医学書院,2010.
- 島田洋一,高橋仁美(編):リハ実践テクニック 骨・関節疾患の理学療法 改訂第2版.メジカルビュー社,2010.
- 椿原彰夫(編著):PT・OT・ST・ナースを目指す人のためのリハビリテーション総論 要点整理と用語解説 改訂第2版.診断と治療社,2013.

MEMO

MEMO

リハビリテーション英語の基本用語と表現
Essential Terms and Expressions for Rehabilitation

2015年 2月 1日	第1版第1刷発行
2022年 8月 1日	第5刷発行

- ■ 編　著　清水　雅子　しみずまさこ
　　　　　　服部しのぶ　はっとりしのぶ

- ■ 発行者　吉田富生

- ■ 発行所　株式会社メジカルビュー社
　　　　　　〒162-0845　東京都新宿区市谷本村町2-30
　　　　　　電話　03(5228)2050（代表）
　　　　　　ホームページ　http://www.medicalview.co.jp

　　　　　　営業部　FAX 03(5228)2059
　　　　　　　　　　E-mail eigyo@medicalview.co.jp

　　　　　　編集部　FAX 03(5228)2062
　　　　　　　　　　E-mail ed@medicalview.co.jp

- ■ 印刷所　株式会社 広済堂ネクスト

ISBN 978-4-7583-0441-2　C3047

© MEDICAL VIEW, 2015. Printed in Japan

- 本書に掲載された著作物の複写・複製・転載・翻訳・データベースへの取り込みおよび送信（送信可能化権を含む）・上映・譲渡に関する許諾権は、(株)メジカルビュー社が保有しています。

- **JCOPY** 〈出版者著作権管理機構 委託出版物〉
本書の無断複写は著作権法上での例外を除き禁じられています。複写される場合は、そのつど事前に、出版者著作権管理機構（電話 03-5244-5088，FAX 03-5244-5089, e-mail：info@jcopy.or.jp）の許諾を得てください。

- 本書をコピー、スキャン、デジタルデータ化するなどの複製を無許諾で行う行為は、著作権法上での限られた例外（「私的使用のための複製」など）を除き禁じられています。大学，病院，企業などにおいて，研究活動，診療を含み業務上使用する目的で上記の行為を行うことは私的使用には該当せず違法です。また私的使用のためであっても，代行業者等の第三者に依頼して上記の行為を行うことは違法となります。